OCN ONCOLOGY CERTIFIED NURSE EXAM:

Comprehensive Test Questions and Detailed Answer Explanations

(+Scenario-Based Questions, Answers With Explanations)

I0430036

BY
MARY BENETT

Table of Contents

1. Introduction

- Overview of the OCN Oncology Certified Nurse Exam

The Oncology Certified Nurse (OCN) exam is a specialized certification designed for registered nurses seeking expertise in oncology nursing. Administered by the Oncology Nursing Certification Corporation (ONCC), the OCN exam evaluates the nurse's knowledge, skills, and abilities related to cancer care.

Exam Content:
The OCN exam covers a wide range of topics within oncology nursing. Key content areas include cancer treatment modalities, symptom management, psychosocial aspects of care, cancer prevention and early detection, survivorship, end-of-life care, and professional performance. This comprehensive scope ensures that certified nurses possess a thorough understanding of cancer care across the continuum.

Eligibility:
Candidates for the OCN exam must meet specific eligibility criteria, including holding a current, unrestricted RN license, having a minimum of one year of experience as an RN in an oncology setting, and completing at least 1,000 hours of oncology nursing practice within the past 30 months. Meeting these requirements ensures that candidates have a solid foundation in oncology nursing practice.

Exam Format:
The OCN exam consists of 165 multiple-choice questions, with 125 questions contributing to the final score. The remaining 40 questions are pretest items used for future exam development. The test is administered in a computer-based format, allowing candidates to receive immediate results upon completion.

Preparation:
Preparation for the OCN exam is crucial, and resources such as review courses, textbooks, and practice exams are recommended. The ONCC provides a detailed test blueprint outlining the percentage of questions dedicated to each content area. This helps candidates focus their study efforts on areas where they may need improvement.

Recertification:
Certification is valid for four years, after which nurses must recertify by meeting continuing education requirements or retaking the exam. This ensures that OCN-certified nurses stay current with advancements in oncology nursing and maintain their commitment to excellence in patient care.

Benefits of Certification:
Achieving OCN certification signifies a nurse's dedication to excellence in oncology nursing. It enhances career opportunities, demonstrates a commitment to professional growth, and instills confidence in both patients and employers regarding the nurse's expertise in cancer care.

In summary, the OCN Oncology Certified Nurse Exam is a rigorous assessment that validates the specialized knowledge and skills of registered nurses in the field of oncology. Certification not only reflects a nurse's commitment to excellence but also contributes to the overall quality of cancer care provided to patients.

- Importance of Certification in Oncology Nursing

Certification in oncology nursing holds paramount importance in the healthcare industry, reflecting a nurse's commitment to specialized knowledge and high standards of care within the challenging field of oncology. Several key factors contribute to the significance of certification in oncology nursing:

1. **Expertise and Specialization:**
   Oncology nursing certification signifies a nurse's advanced knowledge and expertise in the specific field of cancer care. Certified nurses possess in-depth understanding and skills related to cancer treatment modalities, symptom management, and the psychosocial aspects of caring for oncology patients.

2. **Quality Patient Care:**
   Certification ensures that nurses have acquired the necessary skills to provide quality care to patients with cancer. This includes a comprehensive understanding of cancer prevention, early detection, and survivorship, contributing to improved patient outcomes and overall satisfaction.

3. **Professional Development:**
   Obtaining certification demonstrates a commitment to professional development. Oncology nurses who pursue certification are likely to engage in ongoing education, staying abreast of the latest advancements, research findings, and evidence-based practices in cancer care. This continuous learning benefits both the nurse and the patients they serve.

4. **Career Advancement:**
   Certification in oncology nursing opens doors to various career advancement opportunities. Many healthcare institutions recognize and value specialized certifications, and nurses with such credentials often have a competitive edge in job applications, promotions, and leadership roles within oncology departments.

5. **Enhanced Credibility and Trust:**

Patients and their families often seek assurance that their healthcare providers have the expertise needed to navigate the complexities of cancer care. Certification in oncology nursing establishes a level of credibility and trust, assuring patients that they are in capable hands with a nurse who has undergone rigorous training and assessment.

6. **Standardization of Practice:**

Certification sets a standard for oncology nursing practice. It ensures that certified nurses adhere to a set of established guidelines and competencies, promoting consistency and uniformity in the delivery of cancer care across different healthcare settings.

7. **Professional Recognition:**

Achieving certification brings professional recognition and acknowledgment from peers, supervisors, and the broader healthcare community. Certified oncology nurses are often viewed as leaders in their field, contributing to the advancement of nursing practice and the improvement of patient care.

8. **Patient Education and Advocacy:**

Certified oncology nurses are well-equipped to educate patients and their families about cancer, treatment options, and supportive care measures. This advocacy role is crucial in empowering patients to make informed decisions and actively participate in their care.

In conclusion, certification in oncology nursing is vital for nurses seeking to demonstrate their commitment to excellence, advance their careers, and provide high-quality, evidence-based care to individuals affected by cancer. It serves as a benchmark for professional competence and contributes to the overall improvement of oncology nursing practice.

2. Exam Structure and Format

The Oncology Certified Nurse (OCN) exam is a standardized assessment designed to evaluate the knowledge and competence of registered nurses in the field of oncology nursing. Administered by the Oncology Nursing Certification Corporation (ONCC), the exam follows a specific structure and format to comprehensively assess candidates. Here's a detailed breakdown:

1. **Eligibility and Registration:

Before sitting for the OCN exam, candidates must meet specific eligibility criteria. This typically includes holding a current, unrestricted RN license and having a minimum of one year of experience as an RN in an oncology setting. Once eligible, candidates can register for the exam through the ONCC website.

2. Exam Content Outline:

The OCN exam covers a broad range of content areas to ensure a comprehensive evaluation of an oncology nurse's knowledge and skills. The key content areas include cancer treatment modalities, symptom management, psychosocial aspects of care, cancer prevention and early detection, survivorship, end-of-life care, and professional performance. The ONCC provides a detailed test content outline, also known as a blueprint, indicating the percentage of questions dedicated to each content area.

3. Exam Format:

- **Type of Questions:** The OCN exam consists of 165 multiple-choice questions. Out of these, 125 questions contribute to the candidate's final score, while the remaining 40 questions are pretest items used for future exam development.
- **Time Limit:** The exam is time-limited, typically lasting around 3 hours. This includes the time required for a brief tutorial at the beginning.
- **Computer-Based Testing:** The OCN exam is administered in a computer-based format. Candidates can take the exam at designated testing centers, providing a convenient and secure environment.

4. Scoring:

- **Immediate Results:** After completing the exam, candidates receive immediate unofficial results on the computer screen. The official results, including a detailed score report, are mailed to candidates within a few weeks.
- **Passing Score:** The passing score is determined through a standardized process, ensuring fairness and consistency. The passing score may vary slightly from one exam administration to another.

5. Preparation Resources:

- **Test Blueprint:** The ONCC provides a detailed test blueprint outlining the content areas covered and the percentage of questions allocated to each domain. This helps candidates focus their study efforts on areas where they may need improvement.

- **Review Courses and Textbooks:** Numerous review courses, study guides, and textbooks specific to oncology nursing are available to aid candidates in their preparation.
- **Practice Exams:** Taking practice exams allows candidates to familiarize themselves with the exam format and assess their readiness.

6. Recertification:
- The OCN certification is valid for four years. To maintain certification, nurses must meet recertification requirements, which typically involve continuing education and professional development activities specific to oncology nursing. Alternatively, nurses can choose to retake the OCN exam.

In summary, the OCN exam's structure and format are carefully designed to assess a nurse's competence in various aspects of oncology nursing. The computer-based format, immediate results, and detailed content outline contribute to a comprehensive and efficient evaluation process, ensuring that certified nurses possess the necessary knowledge and skills to excel in the specialized field of oncology.

- Types of Questions

The Oncology Certified Nurse (OCN) exam incorporates various types of questions to thoroughly assess the knowledge and competence of registered nurses in the field of oncology nursing. These question types are strategically designed to evaluate a candidate's understanding of diverse aspects of cancer care. Here is a detailed exploration of the types of questions found in the OCN exam:

1. **Multiple-Choice Questions (MCQs):
- **Standard MCQs:** These questions present a stem followed by multiple answer choices, of which candidates must select the correct option.
- **Multiple Response MCQs:** Candidates may be asked to choose more than one correct response from a list of options. This format assesses the nurse's ability to recognize multiple aspects of a given situation.

2. **Case-Based Questions:
- **Patient Scenarios:** Case-based questions present a detailed patient scenario, and candidates are required to analyze the information provided to answer questions related to the diagnosis, treatment, and nursing care involved.
- **Clinical Decision-Making:** These questions assess a nurse's ability to make sound clinical decisions based on a given patient case.

3. **Matching Questions:
- **Column Matching:** Candidates match items from one column to corresponding items in another column. This format evaluates knowledge of associations and relationships between different elements within oncology nursing.

4. **True/False Questions:
- **Statement Verification:** Candidates assess the accuracy of statements related to oncology nursing. This format tests the nurse's ability to discern between true and false information.

5. **Priority-Setting Questions:
- **Ranking or Prioritization:** Candidates may be asked to prioritize nursing interventions or actions based on the urgency of patient needs. This assesses the nurse's ability to make informed decisions in a time-sensitive manner.

6. **Fill-in-the-Blank Questions:
- **Completion Format:** Candidates are required to fill in the blanks in a sentence or phrase. This tests the nurse's knowledge of specific details related to oncology nursing.

7. **Audio-Visual Questions:
- **Image or Audio Interpretation:** Some questions may include images, such as radiographic images or audio clips. Candidates must interpret these visuals to answer questions related to patient care.

8. **Calculation Questions:
- **Dosage Calculations:** Candidates may encounter questions requiring calculations related to medication dosages and administration. This assesses the nurse's proficiency in accurate drug dosage calculations.

9. **Critical Thinking Questions:
- **Clinical Reasoning:** These questions evaluate the nurse's ability to apply critical thinking skills to complex clinical situations in oncology nursing. They often involve analyzing information, making inferences, and selecting the best course of action.

10. **Professional Performance Questions:
- **Ethical Dilemmas:** Candidates may encounter questions addressing ethical considerations and professional conduct in oncology nursing practice. This assesses the nurse's understanding of ethical principles and their application in real-world scenarios.

In summary, the OCN exam employs a diverse range of question types to comprehensively evaluate a nurse's knowledge, critical thinking skills, and ability to apply theoretical concepts to practical situations within the specialized field of oncology nursing. This multifaceted approach ensures a thorough assessment of a candidate's readiness to provide high-quality care to patients affected by cancer.

- Time Allocation

Effective time allocation is crucial for success in the Oncology Certified Nurse (OCN) exam. Candidates need to strategically manage their time during the exam to ensure they can answer all questions within the allotted timeframe. Here's a detailed exploration of time allocation strategies for the OCN exam:

1. **Understand the Exam Structure:
- Familiarize yourself with the overall structure of the OCN exam, including the total number of questions, the time limit, and the distribution of questions across different content areas. This understanding will help you plan your time more effectively.

2. **Time Budgeting for Different Question Types:
- Recognize that different question types may require varying amounts of time. Multiple-choice questions (MCQs) might be answered more quickly than case-based or critical-thinking questions. Allocate time accordingly, considering the diversity of question formats.

3. **Initial Scan and Quick Responses:
- Start by quickly scanning through all the questions to gauge the scope and complexity. Answer the questions you find straightforward and less time-consuming first. This initial pass helps accumulate points efficiently.

4. **Mark and Prioritize:
- If you encounter challenging questions, mark them for review. Prioritize questions based on your perceived difficulty. This allows you to focus on answering questions you find more manageable initially and then revisit the marked ones during the review phase.

5. **Set Time Limits for Each Section:
- Divide the total exam time by the number of sections or content areas. Set time limits for each section to ensure you distribute your time proportionally based on the importance and number of questions in each domain.

6. **Manage Breaks Effectively:
- If the exam allows breaks, use them strategically. Taking short breaks between sections can help refresh your mind. However, be mindful of the overall time limit and don't exceed the allocated break time.

7. **Review and Finalize:
- Once you've completed all the questions, go back to review and finalize your answers. Use any remaining time to revisit marked questions and carefully reconsider your responses. Ensure that you haven't missed any questions or made simple errors.

8. **Avoid Overthinking:

- While critical thinking is essential, avoid overthinking and spending too much time on a single question. If you find a question particularly challenging, make your best-educated guess and move on. Overusing time on a single question can jeopardize your ability to answer others.

9. **Time Management Tools:
- If the exam platform allows, use any available time management tools. Some computer-based exams have a timer or countdown feature. Keep an eye on these tools to gauge your progress and make adjustments as needed.

10. **Practice Time Management:
- During your exam preparation, simulate exam conditions, including time constraints. Practice answering questions within the stipulated time to develop a sense of pacing and improve your ability to manage time effectively during the actual exam.

In conclusion, effective time allocation is a critical aspect of success in the OCN exam. By understanding the exam structure, strategically managing your time, and practicing under timed conditions, you can enhance your ability to navigate the exam efficiently and maximize your chances of success in becoming an Oncology Certified Nurse.

- Scoring and Passing Criteria

The scoring and passing criteria for the Oncology Certified Nurse (OCN) exam are crucial components that determine a candidate's success in achieving certification. Understanding the scoring process and passing criteria is essential for candidates to prepare adequately and navigate the exam confidently. Here's a detailed exploration of the scoring and passing criteria for the OCN exam:

1. **Scoring System:
- The OCN exam utilizes a computer-based scoring system. The scoring process is automated and aims to ensure fairness and consistency in evaluating candidates' performance.

2. **Passing Score:
- The passing score for the OCN exam is determined through a standardized process. The passing score is the minimum level of performance required for a candidate to achieve certification. It is crucial to note that the passing score may vary slightly from one exam administration to another, as it is determined based on the difficulty level of the specific set of questions presented.

3. **Scaled Scoring:
- The OCN exam uses a scaled scoring system. This system adjusts scores based on the difficulty of the questions. Scaled scoring considers the relative difficulty of the questions answered by each candidate, ensuring that the final score accurately reflects their knowledge and competence.

4. **Immediate Results:

- Candidates receive immediate unofficial results on the computer screen upon completing the exam. These results include an indication of whether the candidate has passed or failed. However, these results are unofficial, and the official results, along with a detailed score report, are mailed to candidates within a few weeks.

5. **Score Report:

- The official score report provides a detailed breakdown of the candidate's performance. It includes the overall score and performance in each content area. This information allows candidates to identify strengths and areas for improvement.

6. **Content Area Performance:

- The OCN exam covers various content areas, and the score report specifies the candidate's performance in each of these domains. This breakdown helps candidates understand their strengths and weaknesses, guiding their future professional development efforts.

7. **Pretest Items:

- Out of the total 165 questions on the OCN exam, 40 are pretest items. These questions are not included in the candidate's final score but are used for future exam development. Candidates are not informed which questions are pretest items, so it is essential to approach all questions with equal diligence.

8. **Retake Policies:

- In the event that a candidate does not pass the OCN exam, there are specific retake policies in place. Candidates can retake the exam during subsequent testing periods, but they must adhere to the ONCC's policies regarding eligibility and waiting periods between attempts.

9. **Recertification:

- OCN certification is valid for four years. To maintain certification, nurses must engage in ongoing professional development activities, such as continuing education specific to oncology nursing. Alternatively, nurses can choose to retake the OCN exam as part of the recertification process.

10. **Confidentiality of Scores:

- The ONCC maintains the confidentiality of candidates' scores. Individual scores are not disclosed to third parties without the candidate's consent, ensuring the privacy and integrity of the certification process.

In conclusion, the scoring and passing criteria for the OCN exam are carefully designed to ensure the validity and reliability of the certification process. Candidates should familiarize themselves with the scoring system, understand the passing criteria, and use the detailed score report as a valuable tool for professional growth and development within the field of oncology nursing.

3. Oncology Basics

- Fundamentals of Oncology Nursing

Fundamentals of Oncology Nursing encompasses a comprehensive understanding of nursing care tailored to individuals affected by cancer. This specialty field combines general nursing skills with specific knowledge related to cancer prevention, treatment, and supportive care.

1. Disease Pathophysiology:
   - Nurses must grasp the cellular and molecular basis of cancer, including the stages of carcinogenesis, tumor growth, and metastasis.
   - Understanding the different types of cancer and their unique characteristics is crucial for providing tailored care.

2. Cancer Treatment Modalities:
   - Knowledge of various treatment options such as surgery, chemotherapy, radiation therapy, immunotherapy, and targeted therapy.
   - Understanding potential side effects and complications associated with each treatment is vital for proactive patient care.

3. Symptom Management:
   - Expertise in managing cancer-related symptoms like pain, fatigue, nausea, and psychological distress.
   - Effective communication and collaboration with the interdisciplinary team to address both physical and psychological aspects of symptomatology.

4. Supportive Care:
   - Emphasizing holistic care by providing emotional support to patients and their families.
   - Recognizing the importance of palliative care and end-of-life care, ensuring patients' comfort and dignity.

5. Patient Education:
   - Empowering patients with knowledge about their condition, treatment options, and potential side effects.
   - Promoting adherence to treatment plans and fostering informed decision-making.

6. Survivorship Care:
   - Addressing the unique needs of cancer survivors, including monitoring for late effects of treatment and promoting a healthy lifestyle.

- Supporting individuals in the transition from active treatment to post-treatment survivorship.

7. Communication Skills:
- Developing effective communication strategies for discussing diagnoses, treatment options, and prognosis with patients and their families.
- Sensitivity and empathy are crucial in navigating difficult conversations related to end-of-life care.

8. Research and Evidence-Based Practice:
- Staying abreast of current research and evidence-based practices in oncology nursing.
- Integrating new findings into clinical practice to enhance patient outcomes.

9. Ethical and Legal Considerations:
- Understanding the ethical dilemmas and legal considerations related to cancer care, such as informed consent and patient confidentiality.

10. Continual Professional Development:
- Oncology nursing requires a commitment to lifelong learning to stay current with advancements in cancer care.
- Participating in relevant conferences, workshops, and training programs to enhance skills and knowledge.

In summary, Fundamentals of Oncology Nursing is a dynamic and specialized field that demands a holistic approach, combining technical expertise, compassion, and ongoing professional development to provide optimal care for individuals facing the challenges of cancer.

- Common Types of Cancer

1. Breast Cancer:
- Predominantly affecting women, but it can occur in men.
- Early detection through regular screenings and self-exams is crucial.
- Treatment includes surgery, chemotherapy, radiation, and hormone therapy.

2. Lung Cancer:
- Often linked to smoking, but non-smokers can develop lung cancer as well.
- Divided into small cell and non-small cell types.
- Treatment involves surgery, chemotherapy, radiation, and targeted therapy.

3. Colorectal Cancer:
- Affects the colon or rectum, commonly arising from polyps.
- Screening through colonoscopies helps detect and remove precancerous polyps.
- Treatment includes surgery, chemotherapy, and targeted therapy.

4. Prostate Cancer:
  - Primarily occurs in men and often grows slowly.
  - Early detection through prostate-specific antigen (PSA) testing is crucial.
  - Treatment options include active surveillance, surgery, radiation, and hormone therapy.

5. Ovarian Cancer:
  - Often diagnosed at advanced stages due to vague symptoms.
  - Treatment involves surgery and chemotherapy.
  - Genetic factors may contribute to the risk of ovarian cancer.

6. Skin Cancer:
  - Basal cell carcinoma, squamous cell carcinoma, and melanoma are common types.
  - Ultraviolet (UV) exposure is a major risk factor.
  - Early detection and removal of abnormal skin lesions are key for treatment.

7. Leukemia:
  - Affects blood and bone marrow, leading to abnormal blood cell production.
  - Classified into acute and chronic forms, and further categorized by cell type.
  - Treatment includes chemotherapy, targeted therapy, and stem cell transplant.

8. Lymphoma:
  - Originates in the lymphatic system, including Hodgkin lymphoma and non-Hodgkin lymphoma.
  - Symptoms include swollen lymph nodes, fever, and weight loss.
  - Treatment involves chemotherapy, radiation, immunotherapy, and stem cell transplant.

9. Pancreatic Cancer:
  - Often diagnosed at an advanced stage, leading to a poor prognosis.
  - Treatment may involve surgery, chemotherapy, and targeted therapy.
  - Limited early symptoms contribute to late-stage diagnosis challenges.

10. Bladder Cancer:
  - More common in older adults and often linked to smoking.
  - Symptoms include blood in urine and frequent urination.
  - Treatment includes surgery, immunotherapy, chemotherapy, and radiation.

11. Cervical Cancer:
  - Linked to human papillomavirus (HPV) infection.
  - Regular Pap smears help in early detection.
  - Treatment involves surgery, radiation, and chemotherapy.

Understanding the characteristics, risk factors, and symptoms of these common types of cancer is crucial for early detection and effective treatment. Regular screenings, lifestyle modifications, and awareness can significantly contribute to cancer prevention and improved outcomes.

- Stages and Grading

Stages of Cancer:

1. **Stage 0 (Carcinoma in situ):**
   - Abnormal cells are present but have not invaded nearby tissues.
   - Often considered the earliest stage, and complete cure is possible with appropriate treatment.

2. **Stage I:**
   - Cancer is localized and limited to the organ of origin.
   - Generally, a smaller tumor size with no or minimal spread to nearby lymph nodes.

3. **Stage II:**
   - Tumor growth is more extensive than Stage I but still confined to the primary site.
   - Possible involvement of nearby lymph nodes.

4. **Stage III:**
   - Cancer has spread beyond the primary site to nearby tissues or lymph nodes.
   - Considered locally advanced, requiring aggressive treatment approaches.

5. **Stage IV:**
   - Advanced cancer with distant metastasis to other organs or distant lymph nodes.
   - Typically associated with a poorer prognosis and more complex treatment strategies.

Grading of Cancer:

1. **Grade 1 (Low Grade):**
   - Cells appear well-differentiated, resembling normal cells.
   - Typically slow-growing and less aggressive.

2. **Grade 2 (Intermediate Grade):**
   - Cells exhibit some abnormal features but are not highly abnormal.
   - Moderate growth rate with a moderate level of aggressiveness.

3. **Grade 3 (High Grade):**
   - Cells appear poorly differentiated, significantly different from normal cells.
   - Often associated with faster growth and increased aggressiveness.

Additional Information:

- **TNM Staging System:**
  - Tumor, Node, Metastasis system categorizes cancer based on the size of the primary tumor (T), involvement of nearby lymph nodes (N), and distant metastasis (M).

- Provides a detailed classification for a more accurate prognosis and treatment planning.

- **Histological Grading:**
  - Examines tissue under a microscope to assess the degree of abnormality in cancer cells.
  - Grading systems vary between different types of cancer but generally assess cell differentiation and growth patterns.

- **Clinical vs. Pathological Staging:**
  - Clinical staging is based on pre-treatment assessments, including imaging studies.
  - Pathological staging involves analysis of surgical specimens and provides a more accurate picture after treatment.

- **Importance of Staging and Grading:**
  - Guides treatment decisions by helping determine the most appropriate interventions.
  - Predicts prognosis, allowing healthcare providers to communicate expected outcomes to patients.
  - Facilitates consistent communication among healthcare professionals about the extent and severity of the disease.

- **Evolution of Staging and Grading:**
  - Staging and grading systems continue to evolve with advancements in cancer research and technology.
  - Molecular and genetic profiling play an increasing role in understanding cancer behavior and tailoring treatment.

Understanding the stages and grading of cancer is integral to formulating effective treatment plans, predicting outcomes, and guiding communication between healthcare professionals and patients. Regular updates to these classifications reflect the ongoing progress in cancer research and care.

4. Cancer Treatment Modalities

- Surgery

Surgery plays a crucial role in cancer treatment, serving as a primary modality for various cancers. The goal of cancer surgery is to remove the tumor or as much of it as possible, along with surrounding tissues that may harbor cancer cells. Here's a detailed note on surgery as a cancer treatment modality:

1. **Types of Cancer Surgery:**
   - *Curative Surgery:* Intended to remove the entire tumor and surrounding tissues, aiming for a complete cure.
   - *Palliative Surgery:* Focuses on relieving symptoms or improving the quality of life rather than curing the disease.

2. **Primary Objectives:**
   - *Local Control:* Removing the tumor helps control its growth and prevent it from spreading to nearby tissues.
   - *Prevention:* Surgery can reduce the risk of cancer recurrence by removing precancerous or suspicious tissues.
   - *Diagnostic:* Surgical biopsy helps confirm the cancer diagnosis and determine its characteristics.

3. **Extent of Surgery:**
   - *Radical Surgery:* Involves removing the tumor, adjacent tissues, and sometimes nearby lymph nodes.
   - *Debulking:* Removes a portion of the tumor when complete removal is not feasible, aiming to alleviate symptoms.

4. **Cancer Staging:**
   - Surgery helps determine the cancer stage, crucial for treatment planning and predicting outcomes.

5. **Technological Advances:**
   - *Minimally Invasive Surgery:* Techniques like laparoscopy and robotic-assisted surgery reduce trauma, pain, and recovery time.
   - *Image-Guided Surgery:* Uses imaging technologies like MRI or CT to enhance precision during surgery.

6. **Risk and Complications:**
   - Surgery entails risks such as bleeding, infection, and adverse reactions to anesthesia.
   - Complications can impact organ function or lead to prolonged recovery.

7. **Combination Therapies:**
   - Often combined with other treatments like chemotherapy or radiation therapy for comprehensive cancer management.
   - Neoadjuvant surgery may be performed before other treatments to shrink tumors.

8. **Patient Selection:**
   - Patient factors, such as overall health, play a role in determining if surgery is a viable option.
   - Age, comorbidities, and tumor characteristics influence decision-making.

9. **Postoperative Care:**
   - Recovery involves monitoring for complications, managing pain, and often rehabilitation.
   - Follow-up care is crucial to monitor for recurrence and address any long-term effects.

10. **Challenges and Future Directions:**
   - Addressing the limitations of surgery, such as the inability to remove microscopic cancer cells.
   - Ongoing research explores targeted therapies and immunotherapies to complement surgical interventions.

In conclusion, surgery is a cornerstone in the multidisciplinary approach to cancer treatment, contributing to curative or palliative goals depending on the patient's condition and the characteristics of the cancer. Advances in surgical techniques and combined therapies continue to enhance outcomes and quality of life for individuals facing cancer.

- Chemotherapy

Chemotherapy is a systemic cancer treatment that utilizes drugs to kill or inhibit the growth of rapidly dividing cancer cells throughout the body. This comprehensive note delves into various aspects of chemotherapy as a cancer treatment modality:

1. **Mechanism of Action:**
   - Chemotherapy disrupts the cell cycle, targeting both cancerous and rapidly dividing normal cells.
   - Various drugs inhibit DNA replication, interfere with cell division, or induce apoptosis (cell death).

2. **Types of Chemotherapy:**
   - *Adjuvant Chemotherapy:* Administered after surgery or other primary treatments to eliminate residual cancer cells.
   - *Neoadjuvant Chemotherapy:* Given before surgery to shrink tumors, facilitating surgical removal.

3. **Drug Administration:**
   - Chemotherapy drugs are delivered orally, intravenously, or through intramuscular injections.
   - Intrathecal administration targets cancers in the central nervous system.

4. **Cycles and Courses:**
   - Treatment is organized into cycles with periods of drug administration followed by rest for recovery.
   - The total course duration depends on the type and stage of cancer.

5. **Combination Therapies:**
   - Often used in combinations to enhance efficacy and minimize drug resistance.
   - Combinations may include drugs with different mechanisms of action.

6. **Side Effects:**
   - Common side effects include nausea, fatigue, hair loss, and myelosuppression (decreased blood cell production).
   - Gastrointestinal symptoms, neuropathy, and mucositis are also possible.

7. **Management of Side Effects:**
   - Supportive medications help manage side effects, such as antiemetics for nausea and blood cell growth factors.
   - Close monitoring and proactive interventions are crucial for minimizing adverse effects.

8. **Response Assessment:**
   - Tumor response is evaluated through imaging studies, blood tests, and clinical examinations.
   - Complete response, partial response, stable disease, or disease progression are possible outcomes.

9. **Indications:**
   - Chemotherapy is employed in various cancers, including hematological malignancies (leukemia, lymphoma) and solid tumors (breast, lung, colon).
   - Used as a primary treatment or in combination with surgery and radiation therapy.

10. **Challenges and Limitations:**
    - Drug resistance can develop, limiting the long-term effectiveness of chemotherapy.
    - Non-specific targeting may lead to damage to healthy tissues, causing side effects.

11. **Future Directions:**
    - Ongoing research focuses on targeted therapies, immunotherapies, and personalized medicine to improve treatment precision.
    - Exploration of novel drug delivery systems to enhance specificity and reduce side effects.

In summary, chemotherapy plays a vital role in the comprehensive management of cancer, targeting rapidly dividing cells throughout the body. Despite its challenges and side effects, ongoing advancements in drug development and treatment strategies aim to improve the effectiveness and tolerability of chemotherapy, contributing to better outcomes for individuals undergoing cancer treatment.

- Radiation Therapy

Radiation therapy is a localized cancer treatment modality that utilizes high doses of ionizing radiation to damage or destroy cancer cells. This detailed note explores various aspects of radiation therapy in the context of cancer treatment:

1. **Types of Radiation Therapy:**
   - *External Beam Radiation:* Delivered from outside the body using machines like linear accelerators.
   - *Internal Radiation (Brachytherapy):* Involves placing radioactive sources directly within or close to the tumor.

2. **Mechanism of Action:**
   - Ionizing radiation damages the DNA within cancer cells, preventing their ability to divide and grow.
   - Both healthy and cancerous cells in the treatment field may be affected, but normal cells can often repair damage more effectively.

3. **Treatment Planning:**
   - Precise planning is essential to target the tumor while minimizing exposure to surrounding healthy tissues.
   - Imaging techniques such as CT scans aid in treatment planning and accurate dose delivery.

4. **Fractionation:**
   - Radiation treatment is often administered in fractions (smaller doses over several sessions) to enhance tumor control while minimizing damage to normal tissues.
   - Fractionation allows healthy cells to recover between treatments.

5. **Linear Energy Transfer (LET):**
   - High-LET radiation (e.g., protons or heavy ions) has greater biological effectiveness in killing cancer cells but is often reserved for specific cases due to its complex delivery.

6. **Indications:**
   - Radiation therapy is used in various cancers, both as a primary treatment and in combination with surgery or chemotherapy.
   - It may be curative, palliative, or used to shrink tumors before surgery.

7. **Side Effects:**
   - Acute side effects include skin reactions, fatigue, and temporary changes in organ function.
   - Late effects may occur months or years later and can involve fibrosis, vascular damage, or secondary malignancies.

8. **Quality Assurance:**
   - Rigorous quality control measures are in place to ensure accurate dose delivery and minimize errors.
   - Continuous monitoring and advancements in technology contribute to improved treatment precision.

9. **Technological Advances:**
   - *Intensity-Modulated Radiation Therapy (IMRT):* Adjusts the intensity of radiation beams to conform to the shape of the tumor, minimizing damage to surrounding tissues.
   - *Stereotactic Body Radiation Therapy (SBRT):* Delivers high doses of radiation in a few sessions, suitable for small, well-defined tumors.

10. **Combination Therapies:**
    - Often used in conjunction with surgery or chemotherapy to maximize treatment effectiveness.
    - Neoadjuvant or adjuvant radiation may be employed to enhance overall cancer control.

11. **Challenges and Considerations:**
    - Balancing the therapeutic benefit with potential side effects and long-term complications.
    - Individualized treatment planning considering tumor type, location, and patient characteristics.

12. **Future Directions:**
    - Ongoing research explores innovations like proton therapy, immunoradiotherapy, and radiogenomics.
    - Emphasis on personalized radiation treatment based on genetic and molecular characteristics.

In conclusion, radiation therapy is a fundamental component of cancer treatment, offering precise and localized intervention. Technological advancements, combined therapies, and ongoing research contribute to refining radiation therapy's efficacy while minimizing its impact on healthy tissues, ultimately improving outcomes for individuals undergoing cancer treatment.

- Immunotherapy

Immunotherapy is a groundbreaking cancer treatment modality that harnesses the body's immune system to recognize and eliminate cancer cells. This detailed note covers various aspects of immunotherapy in the context of cancer treatment:

1. **Principles of Immunotherapy:**
   - Immunotherapy stimulates the immune system to recognize and target cancer cells.
   - Enhances the body's natural ability to fight cancer by activating or modulating immune responses.

2. **Types of Immunotherapy:**
   - *Checkpoint Inhibitors:* Block proteins that inhibit immune responses, allowing T cells to recognize and attack cancer cells.
   - *CAR-T Cell Therapy:* Genetically modifies a patient's T cells to express chimeric antigen receptors for improved cancer cell targeting.
   - *Monoclonal Antibodies:* Designed to recognize specific cancer cell proteins, either tagging them for destruction or blocking their growth signals.

3. **Immune Checkpoints:**
   - Proteins like PD-1, PD-L1, and CTLA-4 regulate immune responses; blocking them unleashes T cells against cancer cells.
   - Checkpoint inhibitors have shown efficacy in various cancers, including melanoma, lung, and bladder cancer.

4. **CAR-T Cell Therapy:**
   - Patient's T cells are extracted, modified to express chimeric receptors, and infused back to target cancer cells.
   - Proven effective in certain blood cancers like leukemia and lymphoma.

5. **Monoclonal Antibodies:**
   - Designed antibodies can block cancer cell growth, deliver toxic substances, or enhance immune system targeting.
   - Used in breast cancer (Herceptin), colorectal cancer (Avastin), and others.

6. **Cancer Vaccines:**
   - Stimulate the immune system to recognize and attack cancer cells, often in preventive or adjuvant settings.
   - Prostate cancer (Provenge) and cervical cancer (HPV vaccines) are examples.

7. **Combination Therapies:**
   - Immunotherapy often combined with other modalities like chemotherapy or radiation for enhanced efficacy.
   - Combinations address different aspects of cancer progression and immune evasion.

8. **Biomarkers and Personalized Medicine:**
   - Identifying biomarkers helps predict patient response to immunotherapy.
   - Personalized treatment plans consider the unique genetic and molecular characteristics of the patient's cancer.

9. **Side Effects:**
   - Immune-related adverse events can occur, affecting various organs.
   - Side effects may include fatigue, skin reactions, gastrointestinal issues, and inflammation.

10. **Response Assessment:**
   - Evaluation of treatment response includes imaging studies, blood tests, and monitoring for tumor biomarkers.
   - Pseudoprogression, an initial increase in tumor size before regression, can occur and requires careful evaluation.

11. **Limitations and Challenges:**
   - Response variability among patients and cancer types.
   - Resistance mechanisms may develop, prompting ongoing research to enhance treatment durability.

12. **Future Directions:**
   - Research focuses on identifying new immune targets, refining combination therapies, and overcoming resistance.
   - Advances in understanding the tumor microenvironment and enhancing immune cell infiltration.

In conclusion, immunotherapy represents a paradigm shift in cancer treatment, capitalizing on the body's immune system to combat cancer. With ongoing research, personalized approaches, and combination strategies, immunotherapy continues to evolve, offering new hope and improved outcomes for individuals facing various types of cancer.

- Targeted Therapy

Targeted therapy is a specialized approach to cancer treatment that focuses on identifying and attacking specific molecules or pathways involved in the growth and survival of cancer cells. This detailed note covers various aspects of targeted therapy in the context of cancer treatment:

1. **Principles of Targeted Therapy:**
   - Targets specific molecules critical for cancer cell survival or growth.
   - Designed to interfere with specific aspects of cancer biology while minimizing damage to normal cells.

2. **Types of Targeted Therapy:**
   - *Small Molecule Inhibitors:* Oral medications that enter cells and interfere with signaling pathways or enzyme activity.
   - *Monoclonal Antibodies:* Engineered antibodies that recognize and bind to specific proteins on the surface of cancer cells.

3. **Molecular Targets:**
   - Targeted therapies focus on proteins involved in cell signaling, angiogenesis, DNA repair, and other key processes.
   - Examples include EGFR, HER2, BRAF, and VEGF.

4. **EGFR Inhibitors:**
   - Used in cancers with overactive epidermal growth factor receptor (EGFR), such as lung and colorectal cancers.
   - Examples include erlotinib, gefitinib, and osimertinib.

5. **HER2 Inhibitors:**
   - Target cancers overexpressing HER2, like breast and gastric cancers.
   - Trastuzumab and pertuzumab are examples.

6. **BRAF Inhibitors:**
   - Used in melanomas with BRAF mutations.
   - Vemurafenib and dabrafenib are BRAF inhibitors.

7. **Angiogenesis Inhibitors:**
   - Target blood vessel formation to inhibit tumor growth.
   - Bevacizumab is an anti-VEGF monoclonal antibody used in various cancers.

8. **Resistance Mechanisms:**
   - Tumors may develop resistance to targeted therapies over time.
   - Combination therapies or next-generation inhibitors aim to overcome resistance.

9. **Companion Diagnostics:**
   - Biomarker testing helps identify patients likely to benefit from targeted therapies.
   - Ensures personalized treatment based on the specific molecular characteristics of the cancer.

10. **Combination Therapies:**
    - Targeted therapies often used in combination with other modalities like chemotherapy, radiation, or immunotherapy.
    - Combinations aim to improve treatment efficacy and address multiple aspects of cancer progression.

11. **Side Effects:**
    - Generally, targeted therapies cause fewer side effects than traditional chemotherapy.
    - Common side effects may include skin reactions, hypertension, and gastrointestinal issues.

12. **Response Assessment:**
    - Evaluation includes imaging studies, molecular testing, and monitoring for tumor markers.

- Response criteria may differ from traditional chemotherapy assessments.

13. **Limitations and Challenges:**
   - Resistance development remains a challenge, requiring ongoing research.
   - Side effects and financial considerations may impact treatment feasibility.

14. **Future Directions:**
   - Advances in precision medicine and molecular profiling continue to guide targeted therapy development.
   - Emerging technologies like liquid biopsies enhance real-time monitoring of treatment response.

In conclusion, targeted therapy represents a tailored and precise approach to cancer treatment, addressing specific molecular vulnerabilities within cancer cells. Ongoing research and technological advancements contribute to expanding the repertoire of targeted therapies, offering new avenues for treatment and improved outcomes for individuals facing various types of cancer.

5. Symptom Management

- Pain Control

Pain control is a crucial aspect of patient care, especially in the context of managing various medical conditions, including cancer, chronic illnesses, or postoperative recovery. This detailed note explores the principles, methods, and considerations involved in pain control as a symptom management strategy:

1. **Assessment of Pain:**
- Thorough assessment is essential, considering the nature, intensity, duration, and impact of pain on the patient's quality of life.
  - Pain scales, patient self-report, and observation are utilized to quantify and qualify pain.

2. **Multidimensional Nature of Pain:**
  - Pain is a complex experience involving physical, emotional, and psychological components.
  - Addressing all dimensions is vital for comprehensive pain management.

3. **Types of Pain:**
  - *Nociceptive Pain:* Caused by tissue damage or inflammation.
  - *Neuropathic Pain:* Results from nerve damage or dysfunction.
  - *Mixed Pain:* Combination of nociceptive and neuropathic elements.

4. **Pharmacological Approaches:**
  - *Non-Opioid Analgesics:* Include nonsteroidal anti-inflammatory drugs (NSAIDs) and acetaminophen.
  - *Opioid Analgesics:* Range from mild opioids (codeine) to strong opioids (morphine, oxycodone).
  - *Adjuvant Medications:* Antidepressants and anticonvulsants may enhance pain relief, especially in neuropathic pain.

5. **Route of Administration:**
  - Medications can be administered orally, intravenously, transdermally, or through various other routes.
  - Route selection depends on the type and severity of pain, patient preferences, and treatment goals.

6. **Patient-Centered Approach:**
  - Individualized treatment plans consider patient preferences, cultural factors, and potential side effects.
  - Shared decision-making involves patients in choosing the most appropriate pain management strategy.

7. **Non-Pharmacological Approaches:**
   - *Physical Therapy:* Exercises and modalities to improve function and reduce pain.
   - *Cognitive-Behavioral Therapy (CBT):* Addresses psychological aspects of pain perception.
   - *Interventional Procedures:* Injections, nerve blocks, or implants to target specific pain sources.

8. **Combination Therapies:**
   - Multimodal approaches often combine pharmacological and non-pharmacological interventions.
   - Reduces reliance on high doses of opioids and minimizes side effects.

9. **Palliative Care and Hospice:**
   - Focuses on improving the quality of life for individuals with serious illnesses, incorporating pain control as a central element.
   - Hospice care, in particular, prioritizes comfort and symptom management for those in the final stages of life.

10. **Management of Opioid Therapy:**
   - Requires careful titration and monitoring for potential side effects, tolerance, and dependence.
   - Regular reassessment and adjustments are essential for maintaining optimal pain control.

11. **Potential Barriers and Challenges:**
   - Concerns about opioid misuse and addiction necessitate careful risk assessment.
   - Access to pain medications, regulatory constraints, and stigma surrounding opioid use can be barriers.

12. **Ethical Considerations:**
   - Balancing pain control with the potential risks of addiction and side effects.
   - Respect for patient autonomy and the right to adequate pain relief.

13. **Education and Communication:**
   - Patient and caregiver education on pain management expectations and possible side effects.
   - Open communication fosters a trusting relationship between healthcare providers and patients.

14. **Research and Innovation:**
   - Ongoing research explores novel pain management strategies and medications.
   - Advances in neurobiology contribute to a deeper understanding of pain mechanisms.

In conclusion, pain control is a dynamic and multifaceted aspect of healthcare, requiring a comprehensive and individualized approach. Through a combination of pharmacological and non-pharmacological interventions, patient-centered care, and ongoing research, healthcare professionals strive to optimize pain relief while minimizing potential risks and enhancing the overall well-being of patients.

- Nausea and Vomiting

Nausea and vomiting are common symptoms associated with various medical conditions, treatments, or interventions. Managing these symptoms is crucial to improve the quality of life for individuals undergoing medical care. This detailed note explores the causes, assessment, and comprehensive approaches to the management of nausea and vomiting:

1. **Causes of Nausea and Vomiting:**
   - **Chemotherapy-Induced Nausea and Vomiting (CINV):** A common side effect of cancer treatment.
   - **Postoperative Nausea and Vomiting (PONV):** Occurs after surgical procedures.
   - **Gastrointestinal Disorders:** Conditions like gastritis, peptic ulcers, or gastroenteritis.
   - **Motion Sickness:** Triggered by motion or changes in position.
   - **Medication Side Effects:** Some drugs, including opioids and certain antibiotics, can cause nausea and vomiting.

2. **Assessment:**
   - Thorough assessment includes the frequency, intensity, duration, and triggers of nausea and vomiting.
   - Patient self-report, observation, and clinical evaluation contribute to a comprehensive assessment.

3. **Types of Nausea and Vomiting:**
   - **Acute:** Sudden onset, often related to specific triggers.
   - **Chronic:** Persistent or recurrent over an extended period, requiring more in-depth investigation.

4. **Pharmacological Approaches:**
   - **Antiemetic Medications:** Target receptors involved in the vomiting reflex.
     - Serotonin (5-HT3) receptor antagonists (ondansetron, granisetron).
     - Dopamine receptor antagonists (metoclopramide).
     - NK1 receptor antagonists (aprepitant).
   - **Corticosteroids:** Such as dexamethasone, often used in combination with other antiemetics.

5. **Prophylactic vs. Reactive Treatment:**
   - Prophylactic antiemetics administered before potential triggers (e.g., chemotherapy) to prevent symptoms.
   - Reactive treatment addresses nausea and vomiting once they occur.

6. **Combination Therapies:**
  - Multimodal approaches often involve combining different classes of antiemetic medications for enhanced efficacy.
  - Tailored to the specific triggers and characteristics of nausea and vomiting.

7. **Non-Pharmacological Approaches:**
  - **Behavioral Interventions:** Relaxation techniques, guided imagery, and biofeedback.
  - **Acupressure and Acupuncture:** Can be effective, particularly in certain patient populations.
  - **Dietary Modifications:** Avoiding strong odors and consuming small, frequent meals.

8. **Management of Specific Causes:**
  - **CINV Management:** Prophylactic antiemetics, often in combination, tailored to the emetogenic potential of chemotherapy.
  - **PONV Management:** Prophylactic antiemetics, intraoperative measures, and postoperative strategies.
  - **Gastrointestinal Disorders:** Treating the underlying cause, such as H. pylori eradication for peptic ulcers.

9. **Special Populations:**
  - **Pediatric Patients:** Considerations for age-appropriate formulations and potential psychological factors.
  - **Pregnant Women:** Management considerations, emphasizing safety for both mother and fetus.

10. **Patient Education:**
  - Providing information about potential triggers, management strategies, and when to seek medical attention.
  - Encouraging open communication to address concerns and optimize symptom relief.

11. **Reassessment and Adjustments:**
  - Continuous monitoring for the effectiveness of interventions.
  - Adjustments to treatment plans based on the patient's response and evolving clinical circumstances.

12. **Psychosocial Support:**
  - Nausea and vomiting can impact the emotional well-being of individuals.
  - Psychosocial support, including counseling and support groups, can be integral to holistic symptom management.

13. **Research and Innovation:**
  - Ongoing research explores new antiemetic agents and novel approaches for more targeted and personalized management.

- Advances in understanding the neurophysiology of nausea contribute to innovative interventions.

In conclusion, the management of nausea and vomiting requires a comprehensive and individualized approach, considering the underlying causes, patient characteristics, and potential triggers. Through a combination of pharmacological and non-pharmacological strategies, continuous monitoring, and patient education, healthcare professionals strive to optimize symptom relief and enhance the overall well-being of individuals experiencing these distressing symptoms.

- Fatigue

Fatigue is a common and often debilitating symptom experienced by individuals with various medical conditions, including cancer, chronic illnesses, and autoimmune disorders. Managing fatigue involves a comprehensive approach addressing physical, psychological, and lifestyle factors. This detailed note explores the causes, assessment, and multifaceted strategies for the management of fatigue:

1. **Causes of Fatigue:**
   - **Cancer-Related Fatigue (CRF):** A common side effect of cancer and its treatments.
   - **Chronic Illnesses:** Conditions such as heart failure, rheumatoid arthritis, and chronic kidney disease.
   - **Sleep Disorders:** Insomnia, sleep apnea, or disrupted sleep patterns.
   - **Medication Side Effects:** Certain medications may contribute to fatigue.
   - **Psychological Factors:** Stress, anxiety, and depression can contribute to fatigue.

2. **Assessment:**
   - A comprehensive assessment involves evaluating the onset, duration, and pattern of fatigue.
   - Patient self-report, clinical interviews, and objective measures like the Fatigue Severity Scale contribute to assessment.

3. **Multifactorial Nature of Fatigue:**
   - Addressing physical, psychological, and environmental factors is essential.
   - Recognizing and treating underlying medical conditions contributing to fatigue.

4. **Energy Conservation Techniques:**
   - Balancing activities and rest to avoid overexertion.
   - Prioritizing tasks and breaking them into manageable segments.

5. **Physical Activity and Exercise:**
   - Gradual, tailored exercise programs can improve energy levels.
   - Focus on aerobic exercises, strength training, and flexibility exercises.

6. **Sleep Hygiene:**
   - Establishing consistent sleep patterns and a relaxing bedtime routine.
   - Addressing sleep disorders with appropriate interventions.

7. **Nutritional Support:**
   - Adequate hydration and balanced nutrition contribute to overall energy levels.
   - Dietary adjustments, such as smaller, more frequent meals, may help manage fatigue.

8. **Psychosocial Support:**
   - Addressing psychological factors through counseling, therapy, or support groups.
   - Recognizing and managing stressors contributing to fatigue.

9. **Pharmacological Approaches:**
   - Medications may be considered in certain cases, such as stimulating medications for CRF.
   - Treating underlying medical conditions and adjusting medications contributing to fatigue.

10. **Cognitive-Behavioral Therapy (CBT):**
    - CBT can help individuals manage negative thought patterns and improve coping strategies.
    - Focus on goal-setting, problem-solving, and behavioral activation.

11. **Mind-Body Interventions:**
    - Techniques such as mindfulness, meditation, and yoga can enhance overall well-being and manage fatigue.
    - Integrative approaches promote a holistic mind-body connection.

12. **Occupational Therapy:**
    - Occupational therapists assist in managing daily activities to conserve energy.
    - Recommending assistive devices and adaptive strategies.

13. **Fatigue Management Programs:**
    - Comprehensive programs, often in cancer care, offer a structured approach to fatigue management.
    - May include a combination of exercise, education, and psychosocial support.

14. **Gradual Return to Work:**
    - For individuals experiencing work-related fatigue, a gradual return to work plan may be beneficial.
    - Workplace accommodations and communication with employers are essential.

15. **Reassessment and Adjustments:**
    - Continuous monitoring of fatigue levels and adjusting interventions based on the individual's response.
    - Flexibility in the management plan to adapt to changing circumstances.

16. **Research and Innovation:**
   - Ongoing research explores new interventions and medications to address specific causes of fatigue.
   - Advances in understanding the molecular and physiological basis of fatigue contribute to innovative strategies.

In conclusion, fatigue management requires a multifaceted and individualized approach that addresses the underlying causes while incorporating physical, psychological, and lifestyle interventions. Through collaboration between healthcare professionals and patients, a comprehensive fatigue management plan can significantly improve the quality of life for individuals experiencing this pervasive symptom.

- Anemia

Anemia is a common medical condition characterized by a decrease in the number of red blood cells or a decrease in their ability to carry oxygen. Managing anemia involves identifying and addressing the underlying causes, replenishing red blood cells, and optimizing overall patient well-being. This detailed note explores the causes, assessment, and comprehensive strategies for the management of anemia:

1. **Causes of Anemia:**
   - **Nutritional Deficiencies:** Iron, vitamin B12, and folic acid deficiencies.
   - **Chronic Diseases:** Chronic kidney disease, inflammatory disorders, and certain cancers.
   - **Bone Marrow Disorders:** Conditions affecting the production of red blood cells.
   - **Hemolysis:** Destruction of red blood cells, either intravascular or extravascular.
   - **Genetic Conditions:** Sickle cell anemia, thalassemia, and other inherited disorders.

2. **Assessment:**
   - Comprehensive evaluation includes a detailed medical history, physical examination, and laboratory tests.
   - Blood tests such as complete blood count (CBC), iron studies, and reticulocyte count assist in diagnosing and classifying anemia.

3. **Classification of Anemia:**
   - **Microcytic Anemia:** Characterized by small red blood cells, often associated with iron deficiency.
   - **Normocytic Anemia:** Normal-sized red blood cells, seen in chronic diseases and certain bone marrow disorders.
   - **Macrocytic Anemia:** Enlarged red blood cells, commonly due to vitamin B12 or folate deficiency.

4. **Treatment of Underlying Causes:**

- **Iron Supplementation:** For iron-deficiency anemia; oral or intravenous iron may be prescribed.
- **Vitamin B12 and Folate Supplementation:** For deficiencies associated with macrocytic anemia.
- **Treatment of Chronic Diseases:** Managing the underlying conditions contributing to anemia.

5. **Blood Transfusions:**
 - Reserved for severe anemia or situations where rapid correction is necessary.
 - Risks and benefits carefully weighed, and transfusions are typically administered in a hospital setting.

6. **Erythropoiesis-Stimulating Agents (ESAs):**
 - Medications that stimulate the production of red blood cells.
 - Commonly used in chronic kidney disease and chemotherapy-induced anemia.

7. **Lifestyle Modifications:**
 - Dietary changes to increase intake of iron, vitamin B12, and folate.
 - Encouraging a well-balanced diet to support overall health.

8. **Management of Hemolysis:**
 - Addressing underlying causes, such as autoimmune disorders or hereditary hemolytic anemias.
 - Supportive care with folic acid supplementation.

9. **Genetic Counseling and Screening:**
 - For individuals with hereditary anemias, genetic counseling can provide information about the condition and inheritance patterns.
 - Prenatal screening for couples at risk of passing on genetic forms of anemia.

10. **Monitoring and Follow-Up:**
 - Regular follow-up appointments to monitor response to treatment.
 - Adjustments to treatment plans based on laboratory results and patient symptoms.

11. **Patient Education:**
 - Educating patients about their specific type of anemia, contributing factors, and the importance of treatment adherence.
 - Counseling on lifestyle modifications and dietary choices.

12. **Supportive Care:**
 - Managing symptoms such as fatigue and shortness of breath through supportive measures.
 - Addressing psychological aspects of living with a chronic condition.

13. **Research and Innovation:**

- Ongoing research focuses on developing new therapies and understanding the genetic and molecular basis of anemia.
- Innovations in gene therapy may provide potential curative approaches for certain hereditary anemias.

In conclusion, managing anemia involves a comprehensive and individualized approach, addressing the underlying causes and optimizing overall patient well-being. Through collaboration between healthcare professionals, patients, and support systems, effective anemia management can significantly improve quality of life and prevent complications associated with this common hematologic condition.

6. Supportive Care

- Palliative Care

Palliative care is a specialized medical approach focused on enhancing the quality of life for individuals facing serious illnesses, such as cancer, heart failure, or chronic obstructive pulmonary disease. It aims to provide comprehensive support by addressing physical, emotional, and spiritual needs, ultimately offering comfort and dignity.

1. Holistic Care:
Palliative care embraces a holistic approach, considering not only the physical symptoms but also the psychological, social, and spiritual aspects of a patient's well-being. This ensures a comprehensive and individualized care plan.

2. Symptom Management:
It prioritizes effective symptom management, including pain control, nausea relief, and alleviation of other distressing symptoms. This is achieved through a combination of medications, therapies, and other interventions tailored to the patient's needs.

3. Emotional and Psychosocial Support:
Palliative care professionals, including physicians, nurses, social workers, and psychologists, work collaboratively to provide emotional support. Counseling and discussions about coping strategies help patients and their families navigate the challenges of a serious illness.

4. Open Communication:
Facilitating open communication is a key aspect. Palliative care encourages honest and clear discussions about the patient's prognosis, treatment options, and end-of-life preferences. This fosters informed decision-making and helps align care with the patient's values.

5. Advance Care Planning:
Palliative care includes discussions on advance care planning, ensuring that patients have the opportunity to express their preferences regarding future medical interventions. This may involve creating advance directives or designating a healthcare proxy.

6. Spiritual Care:
Recognizing the importance of spirituality, palliative care addresses spiritual needs and values. Chaplains or spiritual counselors may be involved to provide support in accordance with the patient's beliefs.

7. Family Involvement:

Families play a crucial role in palliative care. Support extends to family members, offering guidance on caregiving, emotional support, and assistance in navigating the complex healthcare system.

8. Care Coordination:
Palliative care involves a coordinated approach with other healthcare providers. This ensures seamless transitions between different levels of care and helps in optimizing the overall care experience.

9. Respecting Dignity and Autonomy:
A fundamental principle of palliative care is respecting the patient's dignity and autonomy. Care is provided with a focus on preserving the individual's sense of self and personal choices.

10. Bereavement Support:
The palliative care continuum extends into bereavement support for families after the patient's passing. This involves ongoing assistance in coping with grief and adjusting to life without their loved one.

In essence, palliative care serves as a vital component of supportive care, emphasizing the patient's well-being beyond the scope of curative treatments. Its multi-faceted approach ensures that individuals facing serious illnesses and their families receive compassionate and comprehensive assistance throughout their healthcare journey.

- End-of-Life Care

End-of-life care, often referred to as hospice care, is a specialized form of supportive care that focuses on providing comfort, dignity, and quality of life for individuals in the last stages of a terminal illness. This holistic approach aims to meet the physical, emotional, and spiritual needs of both the patient and their family during this challenging time.

1. Comfort and Symptom Management:
End-of-life care prioritizes the alleviation of pain and other distressing symptoms. This involves a tailored plan of medications, therapies, and interventions to ensure the patient's physical comfort and enhance their overall well-being.

2. Palliative Approaches:
Similar to palliative care, end-of-life care adopts a palliative approach, emphasizing quality of life over curative measures. The focus shifts from aggressive treatments to interventions that enhance the patient's comfort and dignity.

3. Emotional and Psychological Support:

Recognizing the emotional challenges faced by both patients and their families, end-of-life care provides extensive emotional and psychological support. Counseling, support groups, and resources are offered to help individuals cope with grief, anxiety, and existential concerns.

4. Family-Centered Care:
End-of-life care involves the entire family in the care process. Education and emotional support are extended to family members to help them navigate the emotional and practical aspects of caring for a loved one approaching the end of life.

5. Communication and Decision-Making:
Open and compassionate communication remains crucial during end-of-life care. Healthcare providers facilitate discussions about treatment options, goals of care, and end-of-life preferences, ensuring that decisions align with the patient's values and wishes.

6. Spiritual and Existential Care:
Addressing the spiritual and existential aspects of a patient's journey is integral to end-of-life care. Spiritual counselors or chaplains may be involved to provide support and guidance in accordance with the patient's beliefs.

7. Advance Care Planning and Decision Support:
End-of-life care emphasizes advance care planning, helping patients articulate their preferences for medical interventions and end-of-life care. This includes the creation of advance directives and appointing a healthcare proxy. Decision support is provided to guide families in making difficult choices.

8. Dignity and Autonomy:
Preserving the patient's dignity and autonomy is a core principle of end-of-life care. This involves respecting the individual's choices, promoting independence when possible, and ensuring a comfortable and dignified death.

9. Bereavement Support:
End-of-life care extends into the bereavement period, offering ongoing support for families coping with loss. This may include counseling, support groups, and resources to help individuals navigate the grieving process.

10. Multidisciplinary Collaboration:
End-of-life care involves a multidisciplinary team, including physicians, nurses, social workers, counselors, and volunteers. This collaborative approach ensures comprehensive and coordinated support for the patient and their family.

In summary, end-of-life care serves as a compassionate and comprehensive form of supportive care that honors the dignity of individuals facing a terminal illness. By addressing physical, emotional, and spiritual needs, it aims to enhance the overall quality of life during the final stages of life and supports both patients and their families in coping with the challenges of the end-of-life journey.

- Survivorship

Survivorship care is a distinct phase in the cancer care continuum that focuses on providing support and guidance to individuals who have completed their primary cancer treatment and are living beyond the acute phase of the illness. This phase recognizes the unique challenges and needs that cancer survivors face in terms of physical, emotional, and psychosocial well-being, aiming to enhance their overall quality of life.

1. Follow-up Care and Monitoring:
   Survivorship care involves a personalized follow-up plan to monitor for cancer recurrence, manage treatment-related side effects, and address any new health concerns. Regular check-ups, imaging studies, and laboratory tests are scheduled based on the individual's specific cancer type and treatment history.

2. Managing Late Effects:
   Addressing potential late effects of cancer treatment is a key aspect of survivorship care. This includes managing chronic health conditions, addressing fertility concerns, and monitoring for long-term side effects such as neuropathy or cardiac issues.

3. Emotional and Psychosocial Support:
   Recognizing the emotional impact of a cancer diagnosis, survivorship care provides ongoing emotional and psychosocial support. Counseling, support groups, and resources are offered to help survivors cope with anxiety, depression, and the psychological challenges associated with life after cancer.

4. Health Promotion and Lifestyle Changes:
   Survivorship care encourages health-promoting behaviors and lifestyle changes. This may involve guidance on nutrition, exercise, and smoking cessation to improve overall well-being and reduce the risk of secondary health issues.

5. Survivorship Care Plans:
   Individualized survivorship care plans are developed for each cancer survivor. These plans outline the individual's cancer history, details of completed treatments, and recommendations for follow-up care, helping survivors transition to a post-treatment life.

6. Sexual Health and Fertility Support:
   Survivorship care addresses issues related to sexual health and fertility. Support and resources are provided to navigate concerns about intimacy, relationships, and family planning after cancer treatment.

7. Cognitive Health:

Survivorship care acknowledges the potential cognitive challenges faced by cancer survivors, often referred to as "chemo brain." Strategies for managing cognitive changes and improving cognitive health are incorporated into the survivorship care plan.

8. Financial and Employment Support:

Recognizing the financial strain and potential employment challenges faced by cancer survivors, survivorship care includes guidance on accessing resources, managing medical costs, and addressing workplace issues such as reasonable accommodations.

9. Palliative Approaches:

Palliative care principles may continue to play a role in survivorship care, addressing ongoing symptoms and promoting the overall well-being of survivors. This may involve pain management, fatigue management, and support for survivors dealing with lingering treatment effects.

10. Peer Support and Community Engagement:

Connecting survivors with peer support networks and community resources is integral to survivorship care. These connections provide opportunities for sharing experiences, obtaining advice, and fostering a sense of community among individuals who have faced similar challenges.

In essence, survivorship care recognizes that life after cancer treatment is a unique phase with its own set of challenges and opportunities. By providing personalized and comprehensive support, survivorship care aims to empower individuals to lead fulfilling lives while effectively managing the physical, emotional, and practical aspects of life beyond cancer.

7. Nursing Assessment in Oncology

- Health History

Health history is a crucial component of a nurse's assessment in oncology, providing a comprehensive understanding of a patient's medical background. This process involves gathering detailed information about the patient's past and current health, family history, lifestyle, and psychosocial factors. In oncology, this information is especially vital for tailoring patient-centered care and identifying potential risk factors.

1. **Personal Information:**
   - Obtain basic demographic details such as age, gender, and occupation.
   - Record the patient's address and contact information for effective communication and follow-up.

2. **Chief Complaint and Present Illness:**
   - Document the primary reason for seeking medical attention, including the onset, duration, and progression of symptoms.
   - Identify any associated factors, such as pain, fatigue, or changes in weight.

3. **Medical History:**
   - Gather information about previous medical conditions, surgeries, hospitalizations, and chronic illnesses.
   - Pay specific attention to any history of cancer, treatments received, and responses to those treatments.

4. **Medication History:**
   - Compile a comprehensive list of current medications, including prescription drugs, over-the-counter medications, and supplements.
   - Assess the patient's adherence to prescribed medications and potential interactions.

5. **Allergies:**
   - Document any known allergies, including drug allergies, to ensure the safe administration of medications during cancer treatment.

6. **Family History:**
   - Explore the patient's family history of cancer or other hereditary conditions.
   - Identify any patterns of cancer within the family, as this information may influence the patient's risk assessment and screening recommendations.

7. **Social History:**

- Evaluate the patient's lifestyle factors such as smoking, alcohol consumption, diet, and exercise habits.
- Assess occupational exposures or environmental factors that may contribute to cancer risk.

8. **Psychosocial History:**
- Address the patient's emotional well-being, coping mechanisms, and support systems.
- Identify any history of mental health issues, as cancer diagnosis and treatment can impact a patient's psychological state.

9. **Reproductive History:**
- Gather information related to reproductive health, including pregnancies, childbirths, and menstrual history for female patients.
- Discuss fertility preservation options if applicable.

10. **Review of Systems:**
- Systematically assess various body systems to identify any additional symptoms or potential health issues.

By thoroughly documenting the patient's health history, nurses in oncology contribute to a holistic understanding of the individual, enabling the development of personalized care plans and facilitating effective communication within the healthcare team. This information serves as a foundation for ongoing assessment, treatment planning, and support throughout the cancer care continuum.

- Physical Examination

Physical examination is a vital component of a nurse's comprehensive assessment in oncology, aiming to identify physical manifestations of cancer, assess treatment-related side effects, and monitor the patient's overall well-being. Here's a detailed note on the key aspects of physical examination in oncology nursing:

1. **General Appearance:**
- Observe the patient's overall appearance, noting signs of distress, fatigue, weight loss, or cachexia.
- Assess skin color, hydration status, and any visible abnormalities.

2. **Vital Signs:**
- Measure vital signs including heart rate, respiratory rate, blood pressure, and temperature.
- Frequent monitoring is essential to detect any changes indicating systemic issues or treatment-related complications.

3. **Head and Neck Examination:**
- Inspect the head and neck for any lumps, asymmetry, or abnormal skin changes.

- Palpate lymph nodes, especially in the neck, looking for enlargement or tenderness.

4. **Oral Cavity and Mucous Membranes:**
   - Examine the oral cavity for lesions, mucositis, or other signs of chemotherapy or radiation-related complications.
   - Assess the patient's ability to swallow and communicate any difficulties.

5. **Respiratory System:**
   - Auscultate lung sounds to detect any abnormalities or signs of respiratory distress.
   - Monitor for symptoms such as cough, dyspnea, or hemoptysis, which may indicate pulmonary involvement.

6. **Cardiovascular System:**
   - Assess heart sounds and peripheral pulses, particularly for patients undergoing cardiotoxic treatments.
   - Monitor for signs of fluid retention, edema, or other cardiovascular complications.

7. **Abdomen Examination:**
   - Palpate the abdomen for any masses, tenderness, or organ enlargement.
   - Observe for signs of ascites, a common complication in certain types of cancer.

8. **Neurological Examination:**
   - Evaluate mental status, cranial nerves, motor and sensory functions, and reflexes.
   - Monitor for neurological symptoms such as headaches, seizures, or changes in cognitive function.

9. **Musculoskeletal System:**
   - Assess for any signs of bone pain, fractures, or muscle weakness.
   - Consider the impact of cancer or its treatment on mobility and functional status.

10. **Skin Examination:**
    - Inspect the skin for any lesions, rashes, or changes in pigmentation.
    - Be vigilant for signs of infection, hypersensitivity reactions, or dermatologic manifestations related to cancer treatments.

11. **Genitourinary Examination:**
    - If applicable, assess the genitourinary system for signs of urinary dysfunction or reproductive health issues.
    - Monitor for complications related to specific cancer types affecting these systems.

12. **Peripheral Vascular System:**
    - Check for signs of vascular compromise, such as peripheral edema or impaired circulation.
    - Assess for the risk of thromboembolic events, especially in patients receiving certain cancer therapies.

13. **Functional Assessment:**
- Evaluate the patient's functional status, considering the impact of cancer and treatment on daily activities.
- Collaborate with physical therapists or occupational therapists to address functional limitations and enhance quality of life.

By conducting a thorough physical examination, nurses play a crucial role in early detection of complications, monitoring treatment responses, and providing holistic care to individuals undergoing oncology treatment. Regular assessments contribute to the timely identification of issues, allowing for prompt interventions and optimization of patient outcomes.

- Psychosocial Assessment

Psychosocial assessment is an integral part of a nurse's comprehensive evaluation in oncology, focusing on understanding the emotional, social, and psychological aspects of a patient's experience with cancer. This assessment aims to identify coping mechanisms, support systems, and potential challenges, providing valuable insights for tailoring holistic care. Here's a detailed note on the key components of psychosocial assessment in oncology nursing:

1. **Emotional State:**
- Assess the patient's emotional well-being, identifying feelings such as anxiety, fear, depression, or hopelessness.
- Explore the impact of the cancer diagnosis on the patient's mental health and coping mechanisms.

2. **Coping Strategies:**
- Determine the patient's coping mechanisms and resilience in dealing with the challenges of cancer.
- Identify adaptive coping strategies and assess the need for additional support or interventions.

3. **Support Systems:**
- Explore the patient's social support network, including family, friends, and community resources.
- Assess the quality of support and communication within the patient's social circle.

4. **Cultural and Spiritual Beliefs:**
- Inquire about the patient's cultural and spiritual beliefs, as these may influence coping mechanisms and treatment decisions.
- Respect and integrate cultural and spiritual practices into the care plan as appropriate.

5. **Quality of Life:**

- Evaluate the patient's overall quality of life, considering physical, emotional, and social well-being.
- Discuss aspects such as pain management, symptom control, and daily functioning.

6. **Communication and Information Needs:**
   - Assess the patient's understanding of the diagnosis, treatment plan, and prognosis.
   - Identify preferences for communication style and provide information in a clear, empathetic manner.

7. **End-of-Life Planning:**
   - If applicable, discuss the patient's preferences regarding end-of-life care, advance directives, and goals of care.
   - Facilitate open and honest conversations about expectations and support available during this phase.

8. **Financial and Practical Concerns:**
   - Explore the impact of cancer on the patient's financial situation and practical aspects of daily living.
   - Collaborate with social workers or financial counselors to address financial challenges and connect patients with relevant resources.

9. **Sexual Health and Relationships:**
   - Discuss the impact of cancer and treatment on the patient's sexual health and intimate relationships.
   - Provide information about available support and resources for addressing sexual concerns.

10. **Psychosocial Distress Screening:**
    - Utilize validated screening tools to assess psychosocial distress levels.
    - Regularly monitor changes in distress and intervene appropriately, involving mental health professionals when needed.

11. **Existential Concerns:**
    - Explore existential and meaning-of-life concerns that may arise with a cancer diagnosis.
    - Facilitate discussions on purpose, legacy, and life goals.

12. **Caregiver Assessment:**
    - If applicable, assess the well-being of caregivers and their ability to provide support.
    - Offer resources and support for caregivers, recognizing their role in the patient's care.

By conducting a thorough psychosocial assessment, nurses contribute to the development of individualized care plans that address the unique emotional and social needs of oncology patients. This holistic approach enhances the overall well-being of patients and fosters a supportive healthcare environment throughout the cancer journey.

8. Oncology Pharmacology

- Medications Used in Cancer Treatment

Oncology pharmacology encompasses a diverse array of medications used in cancer treatment, aiming to inhibit or eradicate malignant cells while minimizing damage to healthy tissues. The following categories highlight key classes of anti-cancer drugs:

1. **Chemotherapy Agents:**
 - *Alkylating Agents:* Cyclophosphamide, cisplatin, and temozolomide damage DNA, impeding cancer cell replication.
 - *Antimetabolites:* Methotrexate and 5-fluorouracil disrupt nucleotide synthesis, hindering DNA and RNA production.

2. **Targeted Therapies:**
 - *Tyrosine Kinase Inhibitors (TKIs):* Imatinib, erlotinib, and sunitinib block specific kinase pathways, disrupting signals that promote tumor growth.
 - *Monoclonal Antibodies:* Trastuzumab and rituximab bind to specific proteins on cancer cells, promoting immune-mediated destruction.

3. **Hormone Therapy:**
 - *Selective Estrogen Receptor Modulators (SERMs):* Tamoxifen interferes with estrogen signaling in breast cancer.
 - *Aromatase Inhibitors:* Anastrozole and letrozole reduce estrogen production in postmenopausal women.

4. **Immunotherapy:**
 - *Checkpoint Inhibitors:* Pembrolizumab and nivolumab block immune checkpoints, enhancing the immune system's ability to recognize and destroy cancer cells.
 - *CAR-T Cell Therapy:* Genetically modified T cells target cancer-specific antigens.

5. **Antiangiogenic Agents:**
 - *Vascular Endothelial Growth Factor (VEGF) Inhibitors:* Bevacizumab inhibits angiogenesis, cutting off the blood supply to tumors.

6. **Radiopharmaceuticals:**
 - *Radioactive Isotopes:* Iodine-131 and samarium-153 emit radiation, selectively damaging cancer cells.

7. **Cytotoxic Antibiotics:**

- *Doxorubicin and bleomycin:* These drugs interfere with DNA synthesis or induce DNA damage.

8. **Topoisomerase Inhibitors:**
   - *Topotecan and etoposide:* These drugs target enzymes involved in DNA replication, preventing proper DNA repair.

9. **PARP Inhibitors:**
   - *Olaparib and rucaparib:* These drugs interfere with DNA repair mechanisms in cancer cells, leading to their demise.

10. **HDAC Inhibitors:**
    - *Vorinostat and panobinostat:* These inhibit histone deacetylase, modifying gene expression and inducing apoptosis in cancer cells.

Effective cancer treatment often involves combinations of these drugs or modalities, tailored to the specific cancer type, stage, and patient characteristics. Close monitoring of side effects and adjusting treatment plans accordingly is crucial for optimizing therapeutic outcomes.

- Side Effects and Management

Oncology pharmacology, while essential in cancer treatment, often brings along a spectrum of side effects that can impact patients' quality of life. It's crucial to understand and manage these side effects effectively. Here's an in-depth overview:

1. **Chemotherapy-Related Side Effects:**
   - **Nausea and Vomiting:** Antiemetic drugs such as ondansetron and aprepitant are commonly prescribed.
   - **Fatigue:** Adequate rest, balanced nutrition, and exercise may help alleviate fatigue.
   - **Myelosuppression:** Regular blood tests monitor blood cell counts, and growth factors like filgrastim can stimulate white blood cell production.

2. **Targeted Therapies:**
   - **Skin Rash:** Topical steroids or dose adjustments can manage skin reactions associated with EGFR inhibitors like erlotinib.
   - **Hypertension:** Antihypertensive medications such as ACE inhibitors may be prescribed.

3. **Hormone Therapy:**
   - **Hot Flashes:** Lifestyle modifications and medications like venlafaxine may alleviate hot flashes induced by hormonal therapies.
   - **Bone Density Loss:** Calcium and vitamin D supplementation, along with bisphosphonates, can mitigate bone loss.

4. **Immunotherapy:**
 - **Immune-Related Adverse Events (irAEs):** Corticosteroids like prednisone are often used to manage irAEs such as colitis or dermatitis.
 - **Fatigue:** Adequate rest and symptom management are essential.

5. **Antiangiogenic Agents:**
 - **Hypertension:** Antihypertensive medications are prescribed to control elevated blood pressure.
 - **Bleeding Risk:** Close monitoring and platelet transfusions may be necessary.

6. **Radiopharmaceuticals:**
 - **Fatigue:** Adequate rest and hydration are crucial after receiving radiopharmaceuticals.
 - **Bone Marrow Suppression:** Frequent blood tests and supportive medications are used to manage hematological side effects.

7. **Cytotoxic Antibiotics and Topoisomerase Inhibitors:**
 - **Cardiotoxicity:** Monitoring cardiac function and potential use of cardioprotective agents, such as dexrazoxane with anthracyclines.

8. **PARP Inhibitors:**
 - **Myelosuppression:** Regular blood tests and supportive medications address hematological side effects.
 - **Nausea:** Antiemetic drugs can help manage nausea associated with PARP inhibitors.

9. **HDAC Inhibitors:**
 - **Fatigue and Gastrointestinal Symptoms:** Symptomatic management and dose adjustments may be necessary.

10. **General Considerations:**
 - **Psychosocial Support:** Counseling and support groups can assist patients in coping with emotional and psychological challenges.
 - **Nutritional Support:** A well-balanced diet and nutritional supplements help combat weight loss and malnutrition.
 - **Pain Management:** Adequate pain relief is essential, often achieved through a combination of medications and interventions.

In all cases, open communication between healthcare providers and patients is crucial. Tailoring supportive care to each patient's specific needs improves overall treatment tolerance and enhances the likelihood of successful outcomes. Regular monitoring, early intervention, and a multidisciplinary approach are essential components of managing side effects in oncology pharmacology.

9. Psychosocial Aspects of Oncology Nursing

- Communication with Patients and Families

Communication with patients and their families is a crucial psychosocial aspect of oncology nursing, playing a pivotal role in providing holistic care. Effective communication fosters trust, promotes understanding, and addresses the emotional and informational needs of individuals facing cancer. Here's a detailed note on this topic:

Communication in oncology nursing involves the exchange of information, emotions, and support between healthcare professionals, patients, and their families. It encompasses verbal and non-verbal interactions and is a key component of psychosocial care.

Importance of Communication in Oncology Nursing:

1. **Establishing Trust:**
   - Building a trusting relationship is essential for effective care. Transparent and empathetic communication helps establish trust, making patients and families feel supported throughout their cancer journey.

2. **Information Sharing:**
   - Clear and accurate information about the diagnosis, treatment options, and potential outcomes is crucial. Nurses must ensure that information is delivered in a way that is easily understandable, taking into account the individual's educational background and emotional state.

3. **Emotional Support:**
   - Oncology nurses often serve as emotional anchors. They need to be attuned to patients' and families' emotional needs, providing empathy and support during challenging moments, such as diagnosis, treatment, and palliative care.

4. **Facilitating Decision-Making:**
   - Informed decision-making is empowered through effective communication. Nurses play a key role in facilitating discussions about treatment choices, potential side effects, and end-of-life care, ensuring patients and families are actively involved in decision-making processes.

5. **Managing Uncertainty:**

- Cancer often brings uncertainties. Nurses should help patients and families navigate the unknown by providing realistic expectations, addressing fears, and offering ongoing support.

6. **Cultural Sensitivity:**
   - Recognizing and respecting cultural differences is paramount. Effective communication considers cultural nuances, ensuring that care is provided in a culturally competent manner.

Strategies for Effective Communication:

1. **Active Listening:**
   - Engaging in active listening builds rapport and helps nurses understand patients' concerns. This involves focusing on the patient, clarifying information, and validating emotions.

2. **Empathy:**
   - Expressing empathy fosters a supportive environment. Nurses should convey understanding of the emotional challenges patients and families face, validating their feelings and providing reassurance.

3. **Clear and Simple Language:**
   - Complex medical information should be conveyed in clear and simple language. Avoiding medical jargon enhances comprehension and empowers patients to make informed decisions.

4. **Open-ended Questions:**
   - Encouraging open-ended questions invites patients and families to share their concerns and preferences, promoting a collaborative approach to care.

5. **Non-Verbal Communication:**
   - Non-verbal cues, such as body language and facial expressions, play a significant role in communication. Nurses should be mindful of their non-verbal communication to convey empathy and support.

In oncology nursing, effective communication is the cornerstone of compassionate and patient-centered care. By focusing on trust-building, information sharing, emotional support, and cultural sensitivity, nurses contribute significantly to the overall well-being of patients and their families facing the challenges of cancer.

- Coping Strategies

Coping strategies are essential psychosocial components in oncology nursing, as they help patients and their families navigate the emotional and psychological challenges associated with cancer diagnosis and treatment. Oncology nurses play a crucial role in identifying, supporting, and promoting effective coping mechanisms. Here's a detailed note on coping strategies in the context of oncology nursing:

Coping strategies refer to the cognitive and behavioral efforts individuals employ to manage stress and adapt to challenging situations. In oncology nursing, coping is particularly significant, given the emotional and psychological toll of cancer diagnosis and treatment.

Types of Coping Strategies:

1. **Problem-Focused Coping:**
   - This involves actively addressing and solving the challenges at hand. Oncology nurses can assist patients in problem-solving by providing information about treatment options, managing side effects, and supporting decision-making.

2. **Emotion-Focused Coping:**
   - Emotion-focused coping aims to regulate emotional distress. Nurses can help patients express and process their emotions, offering empathetic listening and facilitating access to psychological support services, such as counseling or support groups.

3. **Seeking Social Support:**
   - Social support is a powerful coping mechanism. Oncology nurses should encourage patients to connect with family, friends, or support groups. Facilitating open communication within the patient's social network contributes to a robust support system.

4. **Mind-Body Techniques:**
   - Techniques such as meditation, mindfulness, and relaxation exercises can alleviate stress and improve overall well-being. Nurses can introduce these practices and collaborate with other healthcare professionals to integrate complementary therapies into the patient's care plan.

5. **Cognitive Restructuring:**
   - Helping patients reframe negative thoughts and beliefs can enhance their ability to cope. Oncology nurses can provide cognitive-behavioral strategies to promote positive thinking and resilience.

6. **Educational Coping:**
   - Knowledge is empowering. Nurses should educate patients about their diagnosis, treatment options, and potential challenges. Well-informed patients are better equipped to cope with the uncertainties of their cancer journey.

Role of Oncology Nurses in Coping Support:

1. **Assessment:**
   - Oncology nurses should conduct thorough psychosocial assessments to identify individual coping styles, stressors, and existing support systems. This information guides personalized care planning.

2. **Education:**
   - Providing information about the emotional aspects of cancer and available coping resources is crucial. Nurses serve as educators, helping patients and families understand the importance of coping strategies.

3. **Supportive Communication:**
   - Open and supportive communication is key to understanding patients' coping needs. Nurses can create a safe space for patients to express their feelings, fears, and uncertainties.

4. **Referral to Support Services:**
   - Collaborating with psychologists, social workers, and support groups can enhance coping resources. Oncology nurses should be proactive in connecting patients with appropriate services.

5. **Promoting Resilience:**
   - Encouraging a positive outlook and fostering resilience is integral to coping. Nurses can highlight and reinforce patients' strengths, fostering a sense of empowerment and control.

In the realm of oncology nursing, coping strategies are integral to promoting the psychosocial well-being of patients and their families. By tailoring interventions to individual coping styles, providing education, and facilitating access to support services, oncology nurses contribute significantly to enhancing patients' ability to navigate the challenges posed by cancer.

- Ethical Considerations

Ethical considerations are paramount in oncology nursing, guiding healthcare professionals in making morally sound decisions while providing psychosocial care to patients and their families. Ethical dilemmas often arise in the complex landscape of cancer care, requiring nurses to navigate issues related to autonomy, beneficence, confidentiality, and end-of-life decisions. Here's a detailed note on the ethical considerations in the psychosocial aspect of oncology nursing:

Ethics in oncology nursing involves making principled decisions that respect the autonomy and dignity of patients, uphold their rights, and prioritize their well-being within the context of their cancer journey.

Key Ethical Considerations:

1. **Autonomy and Informed Consent:**
   - Respecting patients' autonomy is fundamental. Oncology nurses must ensure that patients are fully informed about their diagnosis, treatment options, potential risks, and benefits. Obtaining informed consent involves providing information in a clear and understandable manner, allowing patients to make decisions aligned with their values and preferences.

2. **Beneficence and Non-Maleficence:**
- The principles of beneficence (doing good) and non-maleficence (do no harm) guide oncology nurses in providing the best possible care while avoiding harm. Balancing aggressive treatment measures with the potential for side effects and the impact on the quality of life requires careful consideration.

3. **Confidentiality:**
- Safeguarding patient information is crucial for maintaining trust. Oncology nurses must uphold confidentiality, sharing patient-related information only with authorized individuals involved in the care team. Discussing sensitive information in private settings ensures patients' privacy is respected.

4. **Cultural Competence:**
- Recognizing and respecting cultural diversity is an ethical imperative. Oncology nurses must be culturally competent, acknowledging and incorporating patients' cultural beliefs, values, and preferences into their care plans.

5. **Truth-Telling and Honesty:**
- Truth-telling is essential, but it must be done with sensitivity. Oncology nurses navigate the delicate balance of providing truthful information about the diagnosis and prognosis while considering the patient's emotional well-being. Honest communication fosters trust but requires tact and empathy.

6. **End-of-Life Care and Advance Directives:**
- Discussions about end-of-life care and advance directives are ethically complex but essential. Nurses should engage in open and honest conversations about patients' wishes, facilitating advanced care planning and respecting individual choices regarding life-sustaining interventions.

7. **Psychosocial Support:**
- Providing psychosocial support is an ethical imperative in oncology nursing. Addressing patients' emotional, social, and spiritual needs contributes to holistic care, acknowledging the interconnectedness of physical and psychosocial well-being.

Ethical Decision-Making Frameworks:

1. **Principles-Based Approach:**
- Applying ethical principles such as autonomy, beneficence, non-maleficence, and justice guides decision-making. Balancing these principles ensures a comprehensive and morally sound approach to patient care.

2. **Ethical Decision-Making Models:**

- Utilizing ethical decision-making models, such as the four-step process (assessment, planning, implementation, and evaluation), helps nurses systematically address ethical dilemmas, involving patients and interdisciplinary teams when appropriate.

In the realm of oncology nursing, ethical considerations are integral to providing compassionate and patient-centered care. By navigating complex dilemmas with respect for autonomy, cultural sensitivity, and a commitment to truth-telling, oncology nurses uphold the highest ethical standards, ensuring the well-being and dignity of patients throughout their cancer journey.

10. Professional Practice

- Nursing Standards and Guidelines

Nursing standards and guidelines serve as crucial frameworks that guide and regulate professional practice, ensuring the delivery of safe, effective, and ethical patient care. These standards are developed and endorsed by nursing organizations, regulatory bodies, and healthcare institutions to uphold the quality and consistency of nursing services. Here's a detailed note on key aspects of nursing standards and guidelines:

1. **Professionalism and Ethical Practice:**
   - Nurses are expected to adhere to a high level of professionalism, demonstrating integrity, compassion, and respect for the dignity and rights of patients.
   - Ethical principles, such as autonomy, beneficence, non-maleficence, and justice, underpin nursing practice.

2. **Education and Competence:**
   - Nurses must possess the necessary education, training, and competencies to meet the demands of their specific roles.
   - Continuous professional development is encouraged to stay abreast of advancements in healthcare.

3. **Patient-Centered Care:**
   - Nursing standards emphasize the provision of patient-centered care, involving collaboration with patients, families, and other healthcare professionals.
   - Cultural competence and sensitivity are essential for delivering individualized care.

4. **Safety and Quality:**
   - Nurses are responsible for maintaining a safe environment for patients, colleagues, and themselves.
   - Adherence to infection control protocols, medication safety, and error prevention are integral components of nursing standards.

5. **Communication and Collaboration:**
   - Effective communication with patients, families, and interdisciplinary teams is emphasized in nursing standards.
   - Collaboration fosters seamless healthcare delivery and improved patient outcomes.

6. **Documentation and Record-keeping:**
   - Accurate and timely documentation of patient information, assessments, interventions, and outcomes is a critical aspect of nursing practice.

- Proper record-keeping ensures continuity of care and facilitates communication among healthcare providers.

7. **Legal Responsibilities:**
  - Nurses must be aware of and comply with local, state, and federal laws governing nursing practice.
  - Understanding scope of practice and reporting obligations is crucial to legal and ethical nursing practice.

8. **Advocacy:**
  - Nurses are encouraged to advocate for the rights and well-being of patients, promoting equitable access to healthcare services.
  - Advocacy may involve addressing systemic issues impacting patient care.

9. **Research and Evidence-Based Practice:**
  - Nurses are expected to integrate evidence-based research into their practice to enhance decision-making and improve patient outcomes.
  - Participating in and contributing to nursing research is often encouraged.

10. **Professional Boundaries:**
  - Maintaining appropriate professional boundaries with patients, families, and colleagues is essential for ethical nursing practice.
  - Nurses should be mindful of potential conflicts of interest and ensure objectivity in their interactions.

In summary, nursing standards and guidelines provide a comprehensive framework for the practice of nursing, encompassing ethical, educational, safety, communication, and legal aspects. Adherence to these standards ensures that nurses provide high-quality, patient-centered care in a manner consistent with professional values and responsibilities.

- Legal and Ethical Issues

Legal and ethical considerations are fundamental aspects of professional practice across various fields, including healthcare. Understanding and adhering to legal and ethical standards is crucial for ensuring the well-being of individuals, maintaining professional integrity, and preventing potential legal ramifications. Here's a detailed note on the legal and ethical issues relevant to professional practice:

Legal Issues:

1. **Licensing and Certification:**
  - Professionals must obtain and maintain the necessary licenses and certifications required for their practice.

- Operating without proper credentials may result in legal consequences and professional sanctions.

2. **Scope of Practice:**
- Professionals are legally bound by their defined scope of practice, outlining the specific activities and responsibilities they are authorized to perform.
- Deviating from this scope may lead to legal repercussions.

3. **Patient Rights and Informed Consent:**
- Respecting patients' rights, including the right to informed consent, is a legal mandate.
- Professionals must ensure patients receive adequate information to make informed decisions about their care.

4. **Confidentiality and Privacy:**
- Safeguarding patient confidentiality is a legal obligation.
- Unauthorized disclosure of patient information can result in legal actions and damage to professional reputation.

5. **Mandatory Reporting:**
- Professionals are often legally obligated to report certain issues, such as suspected abuse, neglect, or contagious diseases.
- Failure to comply with mandatory reporting requirements may have legal consequences.

6. **Anti-Discrimination Laws:**
- Adhering to anti-discrimination laws is crucial, ensuring fair and equitable treatment for all individuals.
- Violations can lead to legal actions and damage to professional standing.

7. **Documentation and Record-keeping:**
- Maintaining accurate and complete records is not only an ethical responsibility but also a legal requirement.
- Adequate documentation is essential for continuity of care and legal defense if needed.

8. **Medical Malpractice:**
- Professionals can be held legally liable for negligence or malpractice that results in harm to a patient.
- Having malpractice insurance is often a legal requirement to protect against potential legal claims.

Ethical Issues:

1. **Autonomy and Informed Consent:**
- Respecting patients' autonomy and obtaining informed consent are ethical imperatives.

- Professionals should empower patients to make decisions about their care based on accurate information.

2. **Beneficence and Non-Maleficence:**
  - Upholding the principles of doing good (beneficence) and avoiding harm (non-maleficence) guides ethical decision-making.
  - Balancing these principles ensures the best interests of the patient are prioritized.

3. **Justice and Fairness:**
  - Ethical practice involves promoting justice and fairness in the allocation of resources and treatment.
  - Avoiding discrimination and advocating for equitable healthcare access are ethical obligations.

4. **Truthfulness and Honesty:**
  - Professionals must be truthful and honest in their interactions with patients, colleagues, and the public.
  - Honest communication builds trust and maintains professional integrity.

5. **Conflict of Interest:**
  - Identifying and managing conflicts of interest is an ethical responsibility.
  - Professionals should prioritize the well-being of individuals over personal or financial interests.

6. **Cultural Competence:**
  - Recognizing and respecting cultural diversity is an ethical consideration.
  - Culturally competent care promotes positive outcomes and patient satisfaction.

7. **Professional Boundaries:**
  - Maintaining appropriate professional boundaries with patients and colleagues is an ethical imperative.
  - Respecting personal space and avoiding dual relationships preserves trust and integrity.

In summary, legal and ethical considerations are intertwined in professional practice, influencing decision-making, behavior, and the overall quality of care. Professionals must continually stay informed about relevant laws and ethical guidelines, seeking to strike a balance that ensures legal compliance while upholding the highest standards of ethical conduct in their respective fields.

- Cultural Competence in Oncology Nursing

Cultural competence in oncology nursing is essential for providing high-quality, patient-centered care to individuals facing cancer diagnoses and treatments. Oncology nurses must recognize and respect diverse cultural beliefs, values, and practices to effectively address the unique needs of patients and their families. Here's a detailed note on the significance and components of cultural competence in oncology nursing:

Significance of Cultural Competence in Oncology Nursing:

1. **Diverse Patient Population:**
   - Oncology patients come from various cultural backgrounds, each with distinct perspectives on health, illness, and treatment.
   - Cultural competence ensures that care is tailored to individual preferences and needs.

2. **Communication and Trust:**
   - Effective communication is crucial in oncology care, and cultural competence enhances understanding between nurses and patients.
   - Trust is fostered when patients feel their cultural values are respected and incorporated into their care.

3. **Treatment Adherence:**
   - Understanding cultural beliefs and practices helps nurses address potential barriers to treatment adherence.
   - Culturally competent care promotes collaboration, improving patients' willingness to follow treatment plans.

4. **Health Disparities:**
   - Cultural competence contributes to addressing health disparities by recognizing and addressing social determinants of health that may impact cancer outcomes.
   - Tailoring interventions based on cultural considerations can help reduce disparities in cancer care.

5. **Culturally Sensitive Support:**
   - Oncology nurses play a crucial role in providing emotional and psychosocial support.
   - Cultural competence enables nurses to offer support that aligns with patients' cultural norms and coping mechanisms.

Components of Cultural Competence in Oncology Nursing:

1. **Cultural Awareness:**

- Nurses must be aware of their own cultural biases and be open to learning about diverse cultural backgrounds.
- Cultural self-awareness is foundational for providing respectful and individualized care.

2. **Cultural Knowledge:**
- Acquiring knowledge about different cultural practices, beliefs, and traditions is essential.
- Understanding how culture influences health-seeking behaviors and decision-making aids in tailoring care plans.

3. **Cultural Skill Development:**
- Developing communication skills that respect diverse linguistic and cultural nuances is vital.
- Nurses should be proficient in using interpreters and addressing language barriers effectively.

4. **Cultural Encounters:**
- Actively engaging with individuals from diverse backgrounds enhances cultural competence.
- Experiencing and learning from cultural encounters contributes to more effective and empathetic care.

5. **Cultural Desire:**
- A genuine desire to provide culturally competent care is crucial.
- Cultivating an attitude of curiosity and openness fosters a patient-centered approach.

6. **Incorporating Cultural Beliefs into Care Plans:**
- Integrating cultural preferences into care plans respects the autonomy and values of the patient.
- This includes considering dietary preferences, spiritual practices, and family involvement.

7. **Collaboration with Interpreters and Cultural Liaisons:**
- Utilizing interpreters and cultural liaisons enhances communication and understanding.
- Collaboration ensures accurate information exchange and fosters trust between the healthcare team and the patient.

8. **Educational Initiatives:**
- Ongoing education for healthcare providers on cultural competence is essential.
- Workshops, training programs, and resources can help nurses stay informed and continually enhance their cultural competence.

In conclusion, cultural competence in oncology nursing is integral to delivering patient-centered care in the context of cancer diagnosis and treatment. It involves a combination of self-awareness, knowledge, skills, and a genuine commitment to understanding and respecting the diverse cultural backgrounds of patients. By incorporating cultural competence into their practice, oncology nurses contribute to improved patient outcomes, increased trust, and a more inclusive healthcare environment.

11. Practice Questions: Medical Knowledge

- Multiple-Choice Questions with Explanations

Question 1:

Which of the following is a primary risk factor for developing breast cancer?

A) Age
B) Blood type
C) Height
D) Alcohol consumption

Explanation:
A) Age is a primary risk factor for breast cancer, with the incidence increasing as individuals get older. Other factors, such as blood type, height, and alcohol consumption, may have some association but are not considered primary risk factors.

Question 2:

Which type of leukemia is characterized by an overproduction of immature white blood cells, leading to decreased production of normal blood cells?

A) Chronic lymphocytic leukemia (CLL)
B) Acute myeloid leukemia (AML)
C) Chronic myeloid leukemia (CML)
D) Acute lymphoblastic leukemia (ALL)

Explanation:
B) Acute myeloid leukemia (AML) is characterized by an overproduction of immature myeloid cells, leading to a decrease in normal blood cell production. Chronic lymphocytic leukemia (CLL), chronic myeloid leukemia (CML), and acute lymphoblastic leukemia (ALL) involve different cell types and developmental stages.

Question 3:

What is the primary mode of transmission for human papillomavirus (HPV), a known risk factor for cervical cancer?

A) Airborne
B) Bloodborne
C) Sexual contact
D) Fecal-oral

Explanation:
C) Human papillomavirus (HPV) is primarily transmitted through sexual contact, including vaginal, anal, and oral sex. Airborne, bloodborne, and fecal-oral transmissions are not associated with HPV.

Question 4:

Which anti-cancer drug works by inhibiting the formation of microtubules, disrupting the mitotic spindle, and preventing cell division?

A) Doxorubicin
B) Paclitaxel
C) Imatinib
D) Methotrexate

Explanation:
B) Paclitaxel works by stabilizing microtubules, preventing their disassembly and disrupting the mitotic spindle formation. Doxorubicin, Imatinib, and Methotrexate have different mechanisms of action.

Question 5:

What is the primary goal of radiation therapy in cancer treatment?

A) Targeting cancer stem cells
B) Enhancing immune system response
C) Killing rapidly dividing cells
D) Inhibiting angiogenesis

Explanation:

C) The primary goal of radiation therapy is to kill rapidly dividing cells, including cancer cells. It works by damaging the DNA within cells, preventing them from dividing and growing. Targeting cancer stem cells, enhancing immune response, and inhibiting angiogenesis are strategies used in other aspects of cancer treatment.

Question 6:

Which screening test is commonly used for early detection of colorectal cancer?

A) PSA test
B) Pap smear
C) Colonoscopy
D) Mammogram

Explanation:
C) Colonoscopy is a common screening test for colorectal cancer, allowing the visualization of the entire colon for the detection of polyps or cancerous lesions. PSA test, Pap smear, and mammogram are used for prostate cancer, cervical cancer, and breast cancer screening, respectively.

Question 7:

What is a common side effect of chemotherapy known as "chemo brain"?

A) Fatigue
B) Cognitive impairment
C) Nausea
D) Hair loss

Explanation:
B) "Chemo brain" refers to cognitive impairment, such as memory and concentration problems, which can occur as a side effect of chemotherapy. Fatigue, nausea, and hair loss are also common side effects but are not specifically associated with cognitive impairment.

Question 8:

Which hormone receptor status is commonly assessed in breast cancer patients to guide treatment decisions?

A) Estrogen receptor (ER)
B) Progesterone receptor (PR)
C) Human epidermal growth factor receptor 2 (HER2)
D) All of the above

Explanation:
D) Estrogen receptor (ER), Progesterone receptor (PR), and Human epidermal growth factor receptor 2 (HER2) status are commonly assessed in breast cancer patients to guide treatment decisions. These receptors influence the growth of cancer cells and help determine the most effective treatment.

Question 9:

What is the primary purpose of adjuvant therapy in cancer treatment?

A) Relieving pain
B) Shrinking tumors
C) Preventing recurrence
D) Inducing remission

Explanation:
C) Adjuvant therapy aims to prevent cancer recurrence after primary treatment. It is often administered after surgery or radiation therapy to eliminate any remaining cancer cells and reduce the risk of recurrence.

Question 10:

Which imaging modality is commonly used to assess bone metastases in cancer patients?

A) CT scan
B) MRI
C) PET scan
D) Bone scan

Explanation:
D) Bone scan is a common imaging modality used to assess bone metastases in cancer patients. It can detect abnormalities in bone metabolism, indicating the presence of cancer cells in the bones.

Question 11:

What is the purpose of a central venous catheter (CVC) in cancer patients undergoing chemotherapy?

A) Monitoring blood pressure
B) Administering chemotherapy drugs
C) Measuring oxygen saturation
D) Assisting with breathing

Explanation:
B) A central venous catheter (CVC) is used to administer chemotherapy drugs directly into large veins, allowing for safe and efficient delivery. It also minimizes the risk of irritation to peripheral veins.

Question 12:

Which oncological emergency is characterized by a sudden increase in intracranial pressure?

A) Superior vena cava syndrome
B) Tumor lysis syndrome
C) Spinal cord compression
D) Increased intracranial pressure

Explanation:
D) Increased intracranial pressure is an oncological emergency characterized by a sudden rise in pressure within the skull. It can result from brain tumors or metastases and requires immediate medical attention.

Question 13:

What is the primary purpose of supportive care in cancer treatment?

A) Curing cancer
B) Managing side effects
C) Preventing metastasis
D) Inducing apoptosis

Explanation:

B) Supportive care in cancer treatment focuses on managing side effects and improving the overall well-being of the patient. It includes interventions to alleviate symptoms, provide emotional support, and enhance the quality of life during and after treatment.

Question 14:

Which type of skin cancer is most closely associated with excessive sun exposure?

A) Basal cell carcinoma
B) Squamous cell carcinoma
C) Melanoma
D) Kaposi's sarcoma

Explanation:
C) Melanoma is most closely associated with excessive sun exposure and can arise from melanocytes, the pigment-producing cells in the skin. Basal cell carcinoma and squamous cell carcinoma are more commonly linked to cumulative sun exposure, while Kaposi's sarcoma is often associated with immunosuppression.

Question 15:

What is the primary mechanism of action of monoclonal antibodies in cancer therapy?

A) Inhibiting DNA synthesis
B) Blocking cell division
C) Targeting specific cancer cells
D) Enhancing angiogenesis

Explanation:
C) Monoclonal antibodies work by targeting specific cancer cells or proteins, aiding the immune system in recognizing and eliminating cancer cells. They do not inhibit DNA synthesis, block cell division, or enhance angiogenesis.

Question 16:

Which laboratory parameter is commonly monitored to assess renal function during cancer treatment?

A) Hemoglobin
B) Platelet count
C) Creatinine
D) Liver enzymes

Explanation:
C) Creatinine is commonly monitored to assess renal function during cancer treatment. Elevated creatinine levels may indicate impaired kidney function, which can be a side effect of certain chemotherapy drugs.

Question 17:

What is the primary purpose of a peripherally inserted central catheter (PICC) in cancer patients?

A) Administering chemotherapy
B) Monitoring blood glucose levels
C) Assessing cardiac function
D) Measuring respiratory rate

Explanation:
A) A peripherally inserted central catheter (PICC) is used for administering chemotherapy and other medications. It provides a more stable and long-term access point for intravenous treatments.

Question 18:

Which factor is NOT associated with an increased risk of lung cancer?

A) Smoking
B) Radon exposure
C) Air pollution
D) Physical activity

Explanation:
D) Physical activity is not directly associated with an increased risk of lung cancer. Smoking, radon exposure, and air pollution, on the other hand, are established risk factors for the development of lung cancer.

Question 19:

What is the primary purpose of hormonal therapy in the treatment of prostate cancer?

A) Inducing apoptosis
B) Inhibiting angiogenesis
C) Blocking hormone receptors
D) Enhancing immune response

Explanation:
C) Hormonal therapy in the treatment of prostate cancer aims to block hormone receptors, particularly androgen receptors, to inhibit the growth and spread of prostate cancer cells. It does not induce apoptosis, inhibit angiogenesis, or enhance immune response.

Question 20:

Which type of radiation therapy delivers a high dose of radiation to a precise tumor location using multiple beams from different angles?

A) External beam radiation
B) Brachytherapy
C) Proton therapy
D) Gamma knife radiation

Explanation:
A) External beam radiation therapy delivers a high dose of radiation to a precise tumor location using multiple beams from different angles. Brachytherapy involves placing radioactive sources directly into or near the tumor, while proton

---

Question 21:

Which blood cell type is most commonly affected by myelosuppression, a common side effect of chemotherapy?

A) Red blood cells
B) White blood cells
C) Platelets
D) Hemoglobin

Explanation:

B) Myelosuppression commonly affects white blood cells, leading to an increased risk of infections. Red blood cells, platelets, and hemoglobin may also be affected, but the primary impact is on the white blood cell count.

Question 22:

What is the primary role of the oncology nurse in the administration of chemotherapy?

A) Interpreting radiographic images
B) Providing emotional support
C) Conducting genetic testing
D) Performing surgical procedures

Explanation:
B) The primary role of the oncology nurse in the administration of chemotherapy is to provide emotional support to patients and ensure their comfort during the treatment process. Interpreting radiographic images, conducting genetic testing, and performing surgical procedures are typically outside the scope of nursing responsibilities.

Question 23:

Which term describes the spread of cancer cells from the primary site to distant parts of the body?

A) Metastasis
B) Proliferation
C) Apoptosis
D) Angiogenesis

Explanation:
A) Metastasis refers to the spread of cancer cells from the primary site to distant parts of the body. Proliferation is the rapid growth of cancer cells, apoptosis is programmed cell death, and angiogenesis is the formation of new blood vessels.

Question 24:

Which dietary factor has been associated with a reduced risk of colorectal cancer?

A) High red meat consumption
B) Low fiber intake
C) Adequate calcium intake
D) Excessive alcohol consumption

Explanation:
C) Adequate calcium intake has been associated with a reduced risk of colorectal cancer. High red meat consumption, low fiber intake, and excessive alcohol consumption are generally considered risk factors for colorectal cancer.

Question 25:

What is the primary function of the lymphatic system in relation to cancer?

A) Oxygen transport
B) Nutrient absorption
C) Immune surveillance
D) Hormone production

Explanation:
C) The primary function of the lymphatic system in relation to cancer is immune surveillance. It plays a crucial role in detecting and eliminating abnormal cells, including cancer cells. Oxygen transport, nutrient absorption, and hormone production are not primary functions of the lymphatic system.

Question 26:

Which cancer screening test is recommended for early detection of cervical cancer?

A) PSA test
B) Mammogram
C) Pap smear
D) Colonoscopy

Explanation:
C) A Pap smear is a recommended screening test for early detection of cervical cancer. PSA test is for prostate cancer, mammogram for breast cancer, and colonoscopy for colorectal cancer screening.

Question 27:

What is the primary purpose of intraperitoneal chemotherapy in ovarian cancer treatment?

A) Targeting lymph nodes
B) Inducing apoptosis
C) Directly treating abdominal cavity
D) Enhancing immune response

Explanation:
C) Intraperitoneal chemotherapy in ovarian cancer treatment involves directly treating the abdominal cavity with chemotherapy drugs. It aims to target cancer cells within the peritoneum.

Question 28:

Which type of cancer is most commonly associated with the Epstein-Barr virus?

A) Hodgkin lymphoma
B) Lung cancer
C) Pancreatic cancer
D) Colon cancer

Explanation:
A) Hodgkin lymphoma is most commonly associated with the Epstein-Barr virus. Lung cancer, pancreatic cancer, and colon cancer are not typically linked to this virus.

Question 29:

What is the primary side effect of targeted therapy in cancer treatment?

A) Nausea
B) Hair loss
C) Diarrhea
D) Fatigue

Explanation:
C) Diarrhea is a common side effect of targeted therapy in cancer treatment. Nausea, hair loss, and fatigue are also common side effects but are not specifically associated with targeted therapy.

Question 30:

Which type of breast cancer is characterized by the overexpression of the HER2/neu gene?

A) Triple-negative breast cancer
B) Luminal A
C) Luminal B
D) HER2-positive breast cancer

Explanation:
D) Breast cancer characterized by the overexpression of the HER2/neu gene is known as HER2-positive breast cancer. Triple-negative breast cancer, Luminal A, and Luminal B are other subtypes based on hormone receptor status.

12. Practice Questions: Nursing Skills

- Scenario-Based Questions with Explanations

1. Scenario: A patient with diabetes reports feeling lightheaded. What steps would you take, and why?

2. Scenario: A postoperative patient is experiencing increased pain levels. Describe your approach to assess and manage their pain effectively.

3. Scenario: A patient exhibits signs of respiratory distress. Outline the immediate actions you would take and the rationale behind each step.

4. Scenario: A confused elderly patient refuses to take medication. How would you handle this situation, considering patient safety and ethical considerations?

5. Scenario: A patient with a wound dressing needs to be changed. Explain the steps you would follow to ensure proper wound care and infection prevention.

6. Scenario: You notice a medication error has occurred. What immediate actions would you take to address the situation and ensure patient safety?

7. Scenario: A family member expresses concerns about the care provided to their loved one. How would you handle the situation to address their concerns and maintain effective communication?

8. Scenario: A patient is at risk for falls. Describe the preventive measures you would implement and the rationale behind each intervention.

9. Scenario: A patient is newly diagnosed with a chronic illness. How would you provide education and support to help them cope with the diagnosis and manage their condition?

10. Scenario: A patient complains of nausea after receiving a new medication. What assessments would you perform, and what interventions would you implement to address the patient's concerns?

11. Scenario: A patient is scheduled for surgery in the morning. Explain the preoperative nursing assessments and preparations you would undertake.

12. Scenario: A patient is prescribed multiple medications with different administration times. How would you organize and administer the medications to ensure accuracy and patient compliance?

13. Scenario: A patient has a nasogastric tube in place. Describe the nursing care you would provide, including assessments and interventions to maintain tube patency.

14. Scenario: A patient is experiencing symptoms of anxiety. Outline the nursing interventions you would implement to help the patient manage anxiety and promote relaxation.

15. Scenario: A patient presents with signs of infection. Detail the steps you would take to assess and manage the infection, considering isolation precautions and antibiotic administration.

16. Scenario: A pediatric patient requires a procedure. Describe the techniques and communication strategies you would use to alleviate anxiety and gain cooperation from the child.

17. Scenario: A patient is receiving a blood transfusion and develops signs of a transfusion reaction. What immediate actions would you take to manage the situation and ensure patient safety?

18. Scenario: A bedridden patient is at risk for pressure ulcers. Explain the preventive measures and routine assessments you would implement to minimize the risk of pressure injuries.

19. Scenario: A patient with a history of substance abuse is admitted for a medical condition. Discuss the nursing interventions you would implement to address the patient's unique needs and provide support for recovery.

20. Scenario: A patient is receiving palliative care. Describe the nursing interventions you would prioritize to ensure comfort, dignity, and effective communication with the patient and their family.

Explanations

1. **Diabetes and Lightheadedness:**
   - **Assessment:** Check blood glucose levels.
   - **Intervention:** Administer glucose if low, assess for other contributing factors, and monitor vital signs.
   - **Rationale:** Lightheadedness in diabetes may result from hypoglycemia, requiring prompt correction to prevent complications.

2. **Postoperative Pain Management:**
   - **Assessment:** Assess pain intensity using a pain scale.

- **Intervention:** Administer prescribed analgesics, assess for side effects, and explore non-pharmacological pain relief methods.
- **Rationale:** Effective pain management enhances patient comfort, facilitates recovery, and prevents complications.

3. **Respiratory Distress:**
   - **Assessment:** Evaluate respiratory rate, effort, and oxygen saturation.
   - **Intervention:** Administer supplemental oxygen, position for optimal breathing, and notify healthcare provider.
   - **Rationale:** Timely intervention is crucial to address respiratory distress and prevent hypoxia.

4. **Refusal of Medication by a Confused Patient:**
   - **Assessment:** Assess reasons for refusal and cognitive status.
   - **Intervention:** Use communication techniques, consider alternative administration routes, and involve the healthcare team in decision-making.
   - **Rationale:** Ensures patient safety and respects autonomy while addressing potential cognitive barriers.

5. **Wound Dressing Change:**
   - **Assessment:** Assess wound appearance, pain level, and signs of infection.
   - **Intervention:** Follow aseptic technique, provide pain management, and educate the patient on signs of infection.
   - **Rationale:** Prevents infection, promotes healing, and ensures patient comfort during the procedure.

6. **Medication Error:**
   - **Assessment:** Assess the patient's condition and any immediate effects of the medication error.
   - **Intervention:** Report the error to the healthcare provider and document the incident. Implement any necessary corrective measures and closely monitor the patient.
   - **Rationale:** Timely reporting and intervention are critical to mitigate potential harm and ensure patient safety.

7. **Family Concerns:**
   - **Assessment:** Listen actively to the family's concerns, validate their emotions, and gather relevant information.
   - **Intervention:** Communicate effectively, address concerns transparently, involve the healthcare team if needed, and provide support and education.
   - **Rationale:** Building trust through open communication fosters collaboration and enhances patient care.

8. **Preventing Falls:**

- **Assessment:** Identify fall risk factors, including medical history, medications, and environmental factors.
- **Intervention:** Implement fall prevention strategies, such as bed alarms, non-slip footwear, and regular rounding. Educate the patient and family.
- **Rationale:** Preventing falls is crucial to avoid injuries, especially in vulnerable patient populations.

9. **Chronic Illness Education and Support:**
- **Assessment:** Assess the patient's understanding of the diagnosis and emotional state.
- **Intervention:** Provide tailored education, address emotional needs, involve family members, and encourage self-management.
- **Rationale:** Empowering the patient with knowledge and support enhances their ability to manage the chronic condition effectively.

10. **Medication-Induced Nausea:**
- **Assessment:** Evaluate the timing of nausea in relation to medication administration and assess for other contributing factors.
- **Intervention:** Contact the healthcare provider, consider antiemetic administration, and monitor for any worsening symptoms.
- **Rationale:** Timely intervention addresses medication side effects and ensures patient comfort.

11. **Preoperative Nursing Assessments:**
- **Assessment:** Complete a thorough health history, assess vital signs, verify patient identification, and ensure informed consent.
- **Intervention:** Prepare the patient psychologically, administer preoperative medications, and implement any prescribed preoperative procedures.
- **Rationale:** Comprehensive assessments are essential to identify potential risks and ensure a safe surgical experience.

12. **Organizing and Administering Medications:**
- **Assessment:** Review the medication orders, assess the patient's ability to swallow, and check for allergies.
- **Intervention:** Organize medications based on administration times, use the rights of medication administration, and educate the patient about each medication.
- **Rationale:** Ensures accurate and timely administration, preventing medication errors and promoting patient understanding.

13. **Nasogastric Tube Care:**
- **Assessment:** Assess tube placement, drainage, and patient comfort. Check for signs of complications, such as tube displacement or infection.
- **Intervention:** Administer medications as ordered, secure the tube, and provide oral care to prevent complications.

- **Rationale:** Regular assessments and proper care minimize the risk of complications associated with nasogastric tubes.

14. **Managing Anxiety Symptoms:**
   - **Assessment:** Assess the patient's anxiety level, triggers, and coping mechanisms.
   - **Intervention:** Use therapeutic communication, teach relaxation techniques, and consider pharmacological interventions if needed.
   - **Rationale:** Addressing anxiety promotes patient well-being and can positively impact the overall healthcare experience.

15. **Infection Assessment and Management:**
   - **Assessment:** Assess for signs of infection, obtain cultures if necessary, and identify potential sources.
   - **Intervention:** Initiate appropriate isolation precautions, administer antibiotics as prescribed, and educate the patient on infection prevention.
   - **Rationale:** Early recognition and intervention help prevent the spread of infection and improve patient outcomes.

16. **Pediatric Procedure Anxiety:**
   - **Assessment:** Assess the child's developmental stage, fears, and communication preferences.
   - **Intervention:** Use age-appropriate communication, involve parents, provide distractions, and consider comfort measures.
   - **Rationale:** Addressing pediatric anxiety improves cooperation and facilitates a more positive experience.

17. **Transfusion Reaction Management:**
   - **Assessment:** Recognize signs of a transfusion reaction, including fever, chills, dyspnea, and hypotension.
   - **Intervention:** Stop the transfusion, notify the healthcare provider, provide supportive care, and follow institutional protocols.
   - **Rationale:** Prompt recognition and intervention are crucial to prevent severe complications of transfusion reactions.

18. **Pressure Ulcer Prevention:**
   - **Assessment:** Assess skin integrity, mobility status, and nutritional status.
   - **Intervention:** Implement turning schedules, provide pressure-relieving devices, and educate the patient and caregivers on preventive measures.
   - **Rationale:** Preventing pressure ulcers reduces patient morbidity and improves overall quality of care.

19. **Substance Abuse Patient Care:**
   - **Assessment:** Assess the patient's substance use history, withdrawal symptoms, and mental health status.

- **Intervention:** Provide non-judgmental care, involve addiction specialists, and support the patient in their recovery journey.
- **Rationale:** Addressing substance abuse requires a holistic approach to meet the patient's physical and mental health needs.

20. **Palliative Care Nursing Interventions:**
- **Assessment:** Assess physical symptoms, emotional well-being, and the patient's goals for care.
- **Intervention:** Provide symptom management, facilitate open communication, and support the patient and family in end-of-life decision-making.
- **Rationale:** Palliative care focuses on enhancing quality of life, ensuring comfort, and respecting the patient's dignity and choices. Ooo

13. Practice Exam

- Full-Length Mock Exam with Answers and Explanations

1. **Question:** What is the primary goal of radiation therapy in cancer treatment?

   Answer: The primary goal of radiation therapy is to damage and destroy cancer cells while minimizing harm to surrounding healthy tissues.

   Explanation: Radiation therapy targets rapidly dividing cells, such as cancer cells, by damaging their DNA and preventing further growth.

2. **Question:** What is the role of a nurse in managing chemotherapy-induced nausea and vomiting?

   Answer: The nurse should administer antiemetic medications before and during chemotherapy to prevent or minimize nausea and vomiting.

   Explanation: Antiemetics help control nausea and vomiting by blocking signals to the vomiting center in the brain.

3. **Question:** Why is it essential for oncology nurses to assess a patient's pain regularly?

   Answer: Regular pain assessment ensures timely intervention and effective pain management, improving the patient's overall quality of life.

   Explanation: Untreated pain in cancer patients can lead to physical and psychological distress, impacting their ability to cope with the disease and treatment.

4. **Question:** What is neutropenia, and how does it affect cancer patients?

   Answer: Neutropenia is a condition characterized by a low absolute neutrophil count, making cancer patients more susceptible to infections.

   Explanation: Neutrophils are crucial for the body's defense against infections, and a decrease in their count can increase the risk of serious infections in cancer patients undergoing treatment.

5. **Question:** In the context of cancer genetics, what is the significance of BRCA1 and BRCA2 mutations?

Answer: BRCA1 and BRCA2 mutations are associated with an increased risk of breast and ovarian cancers.

Explanation: Individuals with these mutations have a higher likelihood of developing these specific cancers, and genetic testing can help identify those at risk.

6. **Question:** What is the purpose of palliative care in oncology nursing?

Answer: Palliative care aims to improve the quality of life for patients and their families by addressing physical, emotional, and spiritual needs throughout the cancer journey.

Explanation: Palliative care focuses on symptom management, pain relief, and providing support to enhance overall well-being, not just during end-of-life care.

7. **Question:** How can a nurse assess a cancer patient's nutritional status, and why is it important?

Answer: Nurses assess nutritional status by monitoring weight changes, dietary intake, and biochemical markers. Maintaining adequate nutrition is crucial for supporting the patient's immune system and promoting healing.

Explanation: Cancer and its treatments can impact a patient's nutritional status, potentially leading to malnutrition. Regular assessment helps in identifying and addressing nutritional issues promptly.

8. **Question:** Describe the role of the oncology nurse in educating patients about potential chemotherapy side effects.

Answer: The nurse educates patients about potential side effects, emphasizing early recognition and reporting. This empowers patients to actively participate in their care and promotes timely interventions.

Explanation: Patient education helps manage expectations and ensures proactive measures are taken to minimize the impact of chemotherapy side effects.

9. **Question:** What are the key principles of end-of-life care in oncology nursing?

Answer: End-of-life care principles include promoting comfort, maintaining dignity, facilitating open communication, and providing emotional support to both the patient and their loved ones.

Explanation: The focus of end-of-life care is on enhancing the quality of life, addressing physical and emotional needs, and respecting the individual's wishes.

10. **Question:** How does immunotherapy differ from traditional cancer treatments, and what considerations should a nurse keep in mind?

Answer: Immunotherapy enhances the body's immune system to target and destroy cancer cells. Nurses should monitor for immune-related adverse events and educate patients on recognizing and reporting these side effects promptly.

Explanation: Unlike traditional treatments like chemotherapy, immunotherapy harnesses the immune system's power to fight cancer, requiring unique considerations in monitoring and managing potential side effects.

11. **Question:** What is the significance of a complete blood count (CBC) in monitoring cancer patients undergoing treatment?

Answer: A CBC helps assess the patient's overall health by measuring levels of red blood cells, white blood cells, and platelets. It aids in identifying potential side effects of cancer treatments, such as anemia or leukopenia.

Explanation: Monitoring changes in blood cell counts allows nurses to intervene promptly to prevent complications and adjust treatment plans as needed.

12. **Question:** Explain the concept of "cancer survivorship" in the context of oncology nursing.

Answer: Cancer survivorship encompasses the period after completing cancer treatment, focusing on the physical, emotional, and social well-being of individuals who have survived cancer.

Explanation: Oncology nurses play a vital role in providing ongoing support, survivorship care plans, and addressing long-term effects of cancer and its treatments.

13. **Question:** What is the nurse's role in facilitating advance care planning for cancer patients?

Answer: The nurse assists patients in discussing and documenting their preferences for end-of-life care, ensuring these preferences are communicated to the healthcare team and respected throughout the cancer journey.

Explanation: Advance care planning promotes patient autonomy and helps avoid potential conflicts in decision-making during critical situations.

14. **Question:** How does hormonal therapy contribute to the treatment of hormone receptor-positive breast cancer, and what potential side effects should the nurse monitor?

Answer: Hormonal therapy blocks or lowers the effects of hormones that fuel certain types of breast cancer. Nurses should monitor for side effects such as hot flashes, mood changes, and bone density loss.

Explanation: Hormonal therapy is a targeted approach for hormone-sensitive cancers and requires vigilant monitoring to manage side effects and ensure treatment adherence.

15. **Question:** In the context of pain management, explain the difference between nociceptive and neuropathic pain in cancer patients.

Answer: Nociceptive pain results from tissue damage, while neuropathic pain arises from nerve damage. Oncology nurses assess and differentiate between these pain types to tailor interventions effectively.

Explanation: Understanding the nature of pain helps nurses select appropriate analgesics and interventions, optimizing pain control for cancer patients.

16. **Question:** How does targeted therapy differ from traditional chemotherapy, and what are the common targets for these therapies in cancer treatment?

Answer: Targeted therapy specifically targets cancer cells or their environment, often with fewer side effects than traditional chemotherapy. Common targets include growth factors, receptors, and specific signaling pathways.

Explanation: Targeted therapies aim to interfere with specific molecular processes involved in cancer growth, providing a more precise and less toxic approach.

17. **Question:** Describe the nursing interventions to manage mucositis in cancer patients undergoing chemotherapy.

Answer: Nursing interventions for mucositis include promoting oral hygiene, providing pain management, and recommending specific mouthwashes to alleviate discomfort and prevent infections.

Explanation: Mucositis is a common side effect of chemotherapy, and nurses play a crucial role in minimizing its impact on patients' oral health and overall well-being.

18. **Question:** What is the role of a nurse in supporting a patient undergoing a stem cell transplant, and what potential complications should be monitored?

Answer: Nurses support patients through the stem cell transplant process by monitoring for complications such as graft-versus-host disease, infections, and engraftment syndrome. Education on infection prevention and symptom recognition is paramount.

Explanation: Stem cell transplantation is a complex procedure, and nurses play a vital role in monitoring, managing side effects, and providing emotional support to patients and their families.

19. **Question:** Explain the importance of multidisciplinary collaboration in oncology care, and provide examples of healthcare professionals involved in a cancer patient's treatment.

Answer: Multidisciplinary collaboration ensures comprehensive and coordinated care. Healthcare professionals involved may include oncologists, surgeons, nurses, social workers, and nutritionists, working together to address various aspects of the patient's needs.

Explanation: A team approach enhances the quality of care by considering the diverse aspects of cancer treatment and support.

20. **Question:** Discuss the nurse's role in promoting adherence to oral chemotherapy regimens, and what challenges might patients face in adhering to these treatments?

Answer: Nurses play a key role in educating patients on the importance of adhering to oral chemotherapy regimens, addressing potential side effects, and providing support. Challenges may include medication cost, side effects, and patient misconceptions.

Explanation: Adherence to oral chemotherapy is critical for treatment success, and nurses contribute by fostering understanding, communication, and addressing barriers to adherence.

21. **Question:** What are the key principles of infection prevention for cancer patients undergoing treatment, and how does the nurse contribute to maintaining asepsis?

Answer: Infection prevention principles include hand hygiene, proper central line care, and monitoring for signs of infection. Nurses contribute by educating patients, enforcing aseptic techniques, and promptly addressing any signs of infection.

Explanation: Cancer patients undergoing treatment are often immunocompromised, making infection prevention crucial to their well-being.

22. **Question:** Describe the role of the oncology nurse in assessing and managing cancer-related fatigue.

Answer: The nurse assesses cancer-related fatigue by evaluating its impact on daily activities and providing interventions such as energy conservation strategies, exercise recommendations, and addressing contributing factors like anemia.

Explanation: Fatigue is a common and debilitating symptom in cancer patients, and nurses play a pivotal role in its assessment and management.

23. **Question:** What is the purpose of a central venous catheter in cancer treatment, and how does the nurse care for this device to prevent complications?

Answer: A central venous catheter facilitates administration of chemotherapy and other treatments. Nurses care for it by maintaining sterile technique during access, monitoring for signs of infection, and flushing the catheter regularly.

Explanation: Proper care of central venous catheters is essential to prevent infections and ensure the safe and effective delivery of cancer treatments.

24. **Question:** Discuss the psychosocial aspects of caring for pediatric cancer patients, and how can nurses support both the child and their family throughout the treatment process?

Answer: Nurses address the emotional and psychological needs of pediatric cancer patients by providing age-appropriate explanations, supporting coping mechanisms, and offering resources for the child and their family. Regular communication and involving child life specialists can enhance support.

Explanation: Pediatric oncology nursing involves a holistic approach that considers the unique challenges children and their families face during cancer treatment.

25. **Question:** Explain the concept of cancer survivorship care plans, and why are they important for individuals who have completed cancer treatment?

Answer: Survivorship care plans outline post-treatment follow-up, potential late effects, and wellness recommendations. They help survivors transition back to routine care, empower them to advocate for their health, and facilitate communication among healthcare providers.

Explanation: Survivorship care plans enhance continuity of care, addressing the long-term physical and psychosocial aspects of cancer survivorship.

26. **Question:** What role does genetic counseling play in oncology, and how can nurses support patients considering genetic testing for hereditary cancers?

Answer: Genetic counseling helps individuals understand their risk of hereditary cancers. Nurses provide education, emotional support, and assist in facilitating the decision-making process for genetic testing.

Explanation: Genetic information informs personalized cancer risk assessment and management strategies, allowing for early detection and prevention.

27. **Question:** Describe the potential side effects and nursing interventions for cancer patients receiving immunotherapy.

Answer: Immunotherapy side effects may include immune-related adverse events such as rash, colitis, or pneumonitis. Nurses monitor for these effects, educate patients on symptoms, and collaborate with the healthcare team to manage complications.

Explanation: Immunotherapy enhances the immune system's response, but vigilant monitoring and prompt intervention for side effects are essential for patient safety.

28. **Question:** What is the concept of cancer cachexia, and how can nurses contribute to its management?

Answer: Cancer cachexia is a complex syndrome involving muscle wasting and weight loss. Nurses contribute by assessing nutritional status, promoting adequate caloric intake, and collaborating with a multidisciplinary team for symptom management.

Explanation: Addressing cancer cachexia improves the patient's quality of life and helps maintain physical function during cancer treatment.

29. **Question:** Discuss the importance of communication skills for an oncology nurse, especially when delivering difficult news to patients and their families.

Answer: Effective communication is crucial for delivering sensitive information with empathy, fostering trust, and facilitating informed decision-making. Oncology nurses should be skilled in active listening, providing clear information, and offering emotional support.

Explanation: Clear and compassionate communication enhances the nurse-patient relationship and contributes to the overall well-being of individuals facing cancer.

30. **Question:** How does the concept of survivorship change for individuals with metastatic cancer, and what supportive care measures can nurses provide?

Answer: Survivorship in metastatic cancer involves ongoing treatment and symptom management. Nurses offer support by addressing physical and emotional needs, coordinating care, and providing resources for patients living with advanced cancer.

Explanation: Although metastatic cancer is not curable, survivorship care focuses on optimizing the quality of life and addressing the unique challenges associated with ongoing treatment.

14. Test-Taking Strategies

- Time Management

Effective time management is crucial when it comes to test-taking. Here's a detailed note on how to employ time management as a successful test-taking strategy:

1. **Prioritize and Plan:**
   - Begin by understanding the test format and the allocation of time for each section.
   - Identify the sections where you might need more time based on your strengths and weaknesses.
   - Create a realistic schedule allocating time for each section, keeping in mind the total test duration.

2. **Practice with Time Constraints:**
   - Simulate test conditions during your practice sessions. Set a timer and practice answering questions within the stipulated time for each section.
   - This helps in developing a sense of how much time you can afford to spend on each question and avoids panic during the actual test.

3. **Divide Your Time Effectively:**
   - Break down the time for each section into smaller intervals for individual questions.
   - Allot more time to questions that carry higher marks but ensure that you don't spend an excessive amount of time on a single question.

4. **Skip and Return Strategy:**
   - If you encounter a challenging question, don't get stuck. Quickly move on to the next one.
   - Flag the challenging questions and return to them later if time permits. This ensures that you don't miss out on easier questions due to time constraints.

5. **Monitor Your Pace:**
   - Keep an eye on the clock periodically to ensure you are on track.
   - If you notice you're spending too much time on a particular section, adjust your pace accordingly to ensure you complete the entire test.

6. **Budget Time for Review:**
   - Reserve some time at the end to review your answers. This can help catch any careless mistakes and ensure you haven't overlooked any questions.

7. **Stay Calm and Focused:**
   - Manage test anxiety by staying calm and focused. Panic can lead to poor time management.
   - Take a few deep breaths if needed and remind yourself of your time allocation plan.

8. **Be Mindful of Marking Scheme:**
   - Understand how points are awarded for correct answers and whether there are penalties for incorrect ones.
   - Adjust your strategy accordingly, for instance, if there's no penalty for guessing, it might be worth taking educated guesses if you're running out of time.

9. **Build Endurance:**
   - Develop the endurance to maintain concentration throughout the entire test duration.
   - Gradually increase the length of your practice sessions to build mental stamina.

10. **Reflect and Adjust:**
   - After each practice test, reflect on your time management. Identify areas where you struggled and adjust your strategy accordingly for the next practice session.

By incorporating these strategies into your test preparation, you can optimize your time management skills and increase your chances of success during the actual exam.

- Approaches to Answering Different Question Types

Successfully answering different question types requires a strategic approach. Here's a detailed note on approaches to answering various question types as a test-taking strategy:

1. **Multiple Choice Questions (MCQs):**
   - **Read Carefully:** Pay attention to keywords and nuances in the question.
   - **Elimination Technique:** Rule out obviously incorrect options to narrow down your choices.
   - **Consider All Options:** Even if you think you've found the correct answer early on, review all options before finalizing your choice.

2. **True/False Questions:**
   - **Be Precise:** A single word can change the statement's meaning. Read carefully.
   - **Beware of Absolutes:** Words like "always" or "never" in a statement might signal a false answer.

3. **Short Answer Questions:**
   - **Clarity is Key:** Clearly and concisely provide the required information.
   - **Answer the Question Asked:** Ensure your response directly addresses what the question is asking.

4. **Essay Questions:**

- **Plan Your Response:** Spend a few minutes outlining your key points before starting to write.
   - **Stay Focused:** Stick to the main topic and avoid unnecessary details.
   - **Organize Your Thoughts:** Use paragraphs to structure your essay, making it easier for the reader to follow.

5. **Matching Questions:**
   - **Read All Options First:** Before making matches, review all the choices to make more informed pairings.
   - **Elimination Method:** Eliminate obviously incorrect matches to narrow down your options.

6. **Fill in the Blank Questions:**
   - **Context Matters:** Consider the context of the sentence to determine the appropriate answer.
   - **Grammar and Syntax:** Ensure your response fits grammatically within the sentence.

7. **Numeric Answer Questions:**
   - **Check Units:** Confirm that your numerical answer is in the correct units, if applicable.
   - **Estimation:** If permitted, consider estimating the answer to quickly eliminate unlikely options.

8. **Diagram-Based Questions:**
   - **Label Clearly:** If required to label diagrams, ensure clarity in your labeling.
   - **Understand Relationships:** Analyze the relationships between elements in the diagram before answering questions about it.

9. **Critical Thinking Questions:**
   - **Evaluate Arguments:** Analyze the provided information critically before forming your response.
   - **Support with Evidence:** If asked to provide reasoning, back up your answers with relevant evidence or examples.

10. **Experimental/Scenario-Based Questions:**
   - **Understand the Scenario:** Familiarize yourself with the given situation or experiment.
   - **Apply Knowledge:** Use your understanding of the subject matter to answer questions related to the scenario.

Adapting your approach based on the question type is crucial for success in various types of exams. Practice with diverse question formats to refine these strategies and improve your overall test-taking skills.

15. Conclusion

- Final Tips for Exam Success

1. **Comprehensive Review:**
   - Ensure you have a comprehensive understanding of oncology nursing principles, including cancer types, treatments, and symptom management.
   - Review key topics such as chemotherapy administration, side effect management, and patient education.

2. **Stay Updated:**
   - Keep abreast of the latest developments in oncology nursing by staying updated on recent research, treatment modalities, and advancements in the field.

3. **Practice with Mock Exams:**
   - Utilize practice exams to simulate the actual testing environment. This helps in familiarizing yourself with the format and time constraints of the exam.

4. **Identify Weak Areas:**
   - Assess your strengths and weaknesses in different content areas. Allocate more study time to areas where you feel less confident and seek additional resources for clarification.

5. **Create a Study Schedule:**
   - Develop a realistic study schedule that allows for thorough coverage of all relevant topics. Break down the material into manageable sections and stick to your timetable.

6. **Interactive Learning:**
   - Engage in interactive learning methods such as group discussions, case studies, or study groups. Explaining concepts to others can enhance your understanding.

7. **Use Mnemonics and Memory Aids:**
   - Employ mnemonic devices and memory aids to remember complex information, drug names, and classification systems.

8. **Focus on Critical Thinking:**
   - Oncology nursing exams often require critical thinking skills. Practice analyzing patient scenarios, prioritizing interventions, and making sound clinical judgments.

9. **Review Guidelines and Protocols:**
   - Familiarize yourself with relevant oncology nursing guidelines and protocols. Understand the standard procedures for patient care, safety measures, and ethical considerations.

10. **Take Care of Yourself:**
- Prioritize self-care, including sufficient sleep, a balanced diet, and regular breaks during study sessions. Maintaining your well-being is crucial for optimal cognitive function.

11. **Ask for Support:**
- If you encounter challenging concepts or have questions, don't hesitate to seek support from instructors, colleagues, or online communities specializing in oncology nursing.

12. **Mindful Test-Taking:**
- During the exam, read questions carefully, consider all answer choices, and trust your knowledge. Manage your time effectively to ensure you address all questions.

Remember, success in the Oncology Certified Nursing exam requires a combination of knowledge, critical thinking, and effective test-taking strategies.

- Resources for Further Study

1. **Textbooks:**
- **"Oncology Nursing: Scope and Standards of Practice"** - Published by the Oncology Nursing Society (ONS), this textbook provides a comprehensive overview of the standards and scope of practice in oncology nursing.

- **"Cancer Nursing: Principles and Practice"** - A widely used textbook covering essential principles and practices in cancer nursing, offering in-depth insights into various aspects of oncology care.

2. **Oncology Nursing Journals:**
- **Oncology Nursing Forum (ONF):** Published by the ONS, ONF is a peer-reviewed journal covering a wide range of topics in oncology nursing, including research articles, case studies, and clinical updates.

- **Cancer Nursing:** Another reputable journal that publishes research articles, reviews, and case studies in the field of cancer nursing.

3. **Oncology Nursing Society (ONS):**
- The ONS offers various resources, including webinars, conferences, and educational materials. Consider becoming a member to access exclusive content, networking opportunities, and continuing education resources.

4. **Online Courses:**

- Platforms like **Oncology Nursing Certification Corporation (ONCC)** provide online courses specifically designed for nurses preparing for certification exams. These courses cover various topics in oncology nursing and often include practice questions.

- **Coursera and Khan Academy:** These platforms may offer courses related to oncology nursing. Check for relevant courses on cancer care, symptom management, and patient education.

5. **Review Books:**
- **"OCN Exam Secrets Study Guide"** - This comprehensive review book includes practice questions, detailed explanations, and test-taking strategies for the Oncology Certified Nursing (OCN) exam.

- **"Certified Pediatric Hematology Oncology Nurse (CPHON) Review Manual"** - Ideal for nurses specializing in pediatric oncology, this review manual covers key topics for the CPHON exam.

6. **Clinical Guidelines and Protocols:**
- Familiarize yourself with guidelines from reputable organizations such as the **National Comprehensive Cancer Network (NCCN)**. These guidelines provide evidence-based recommendations for cancer care and can be valuable for exam preparation.

7. **Podcasts and Webinars:**
- Explore oncology nursing podcasts and webinars that discuss current trends, case studies, and expert interviews. These can provide a convenient way to stay updated on the latest advancements in the field.

8. **Simulation and Case Studies:**
- Utilize simulation scenarios and case studies to enhance your critical thinking skills. Resources like the **ONS Learning Center** may offer interactive case studies and simulations.

9. **Networking and Conferences:**
- Attend oncology nursing conferences to network with professionals, learn from experts, and stay updated on the latest research and practices. The ONS Annual Congress is a prominent event in this regard.

10. **Professional Nursing Organizations:**
- Joining professional organizations beyond ONS, such as the **American Society of Clinical Oncology (ASCO)**, can broaden your exposure to resources, networking, and educational opportunities.

Remember to tailor your study plan based on your specific needs and exam requirements. Integrating a variety of resources will provide a well-rounded understanding of oncology nursing. **Good luck with your further studies!**